Health and
biomedical information
in Europe

World Health Organization
Regional Office for Europe
Copenhagen

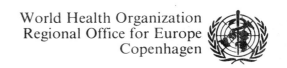

Public Health in Europe 27

Health and biomedical information in Europe

Paul Weiss

Director
Institute for Scientific Information in Medicine
Berlin, German Democratic Republic

ICP/HBI 001/s01

WEISS, Paul
World Health Organization
Regional Office for Europe
Health and biomedical information in Europe
Copenhagen: WHO Regional Office for Europe, 1986
Public Health in Europe 27
      Documentation — Health — Libraries, medical —
      Automatic data processing — Information
      systems — Health services/Organization and
      administration — WHO Regional Office for
      Europe

ISBN 92 890 1163 7
ISSN 0300-4880

PRINTED IN DENMARK

CONTENTS

Preface

In health, as in most areas of development, information is increasingly recognized as an essential tool. Health information can be statistical, providing data on quantitative trends in a country or region; it can also be the integration of statistics, analysis, and description of situations in one or more areas, presented in such a way that readers can make immediate use of it.

The last few years have witnessed an impressive surge in the amount of information available in the areas of biomedical research and clinical medicine, and a corresponding improvement in the use of this information by clinicians and academic investigators. In the field of health management, however, the accumulation of data has not been accompanied by a corresponding increase in the availability and usefulness of information and its utilization by health administrators. Among the targets jointly defined by the Member States of the WHO European Region towards the achievement of health for all by the year 2000, target 35 states: "Before 1990, Member States should have health information systems capable of supporting their national strategies for health for all".

An earlier publication of this Office "Information systems for health services" (Public Health in Europe No. 13) described and discussed the statistical information services in the Region. Professor P. Weiss, Director of the Institute for Scientific Information in Medicine, Berlin, German Democratic Republic, has undertaken for the Regional Office a survey of the "other half" of information, and provides us in the following pages with a review of the general situation in the Region and with specific descriptions of the situation in selected countries. This review has already been put to use in reorienting the documentation services of the Regional Office towards a more active provision of information.

In April 1985, WHO organized in Berlin an initial meeting of institutions responsible for the provision of documentation to health authorities, on the topic "Provision of information and documentation for health management", which recommended that an effort be made towards a better use of the health documentation services available in the Region. The fact that this same topic is to be discussed at the First European Conference of Medical Librarians (Brussels, October 1986) is a heartening sign that health documentation units increasingly see one of their roles as that of actively providing analysed material for immediate use by decision-makers. Our wish is that this book may promote a better understanding between providers and users of information in the service of health for the Region.

Copenhagen, April 1986   J.-P. Jardel

Director
Programme Management

Author's introduction

I wrote this book as a consultant to the WHO Regional Office for Europe in the latter part of 1983. It outlines the present needs for biomedical information in Europe and describes services and networks available for the information of health personnel in the main areas of the Region. I updated my previous experience of this subject by visits to Denmark, France, the Federal Republic of Germany, Italy, Switzerland and the United Kingdom. My knowledge of the problems of health information in the countries of Eastern Europe that collaborate in the Council for Mutual Economic Assistance (CMEA) complemented this experience. I concentrated on the problems of information for health personnel not working in research or hospitals, with special emphasis on two categories of health worker: (a) workers in primary health care; and (b) managers of health programmes and health planners.

Relevant information and documentation are necessary for the proper management of health services at national or regional level, and in the day-to-day management activities of primary health care. The increasing use of on-line data bases, for example, shows how clinical and medical research needs facilities for the retrieval and acquisition of information. In management and primary health care, information and documentation are often inadequate. One reason for this inadequacy is that the material available is presented in a form that people cannot readily use. They most frequently complain that judgement on the quality of the information is lacking. Other problems include lack of legibility, when texts are too long, too abstruse or otherwise unclear, and the fact that health personnel cannot distil available material into a form useful to them in health planning or in primary health care. In addition, the potential user is often not even aware of deficiencies in his or her information.

Improvement of the quality of medical and health care, and in the management of public health, requires the efficient use of existing knowledge. This efficiency will need the cooperation of both partners in the process of presenting and using information: the users learning how better to use the different information sources and documentation services, and the generators and providers adapting their services to the specific information needs of the users.

1

This book is intended for those who believe in the importance of supplying adequate information to people who plan and provide health services, in the hope that improved access to, and use of, information will contribute to better health for the peoples of Europe.

I wish to thank the numerous people who have assisted me in the countries described, in the WHO Regional Office for Europe and at the Institut für Wissenschaftsinformation in der Medizin during the preparation of this book.

Scientific information in medicine: general situation, problems and trends

The Information Explosion — The New Great Flood?

"Of making many books there is no end." "One of the diseases of this age is the multiplicity of books; they doth so overcharge the world that it is not able to digest the abundance of idle matter that is every day hatched and brought forward into the world." Both statements could describe current scientific literature, but both are old complaints. The first is from the Bible (Ecclesiastes 12: 12) and B. Rich, who lived from 1540 to 1617, made the second.

Some 8–10 million scientific and technical documents are now published annually, among them 75 000 books and 300 000 patents (1,2), and 6–7 thousand scientific articles are written each day (3). The existence of 84 000 biomedical journals was reported at the meeting of the Council of Biology Editors in Boston in 1981 (4). Other enumerations of biomedical journals are lower but still impressive (5):

Year	Number of publications
1910	1 000
1930	1 500
1950	4 000
1970	14 000
1980	20 000

Although the number of publications continues to increase, for every three new journals born an old one dies (6).

These estimated figures can lead one to speculate about future developments. For example, if the number of publications continues to grow at its present rate, in 200 years books will arrive at libraries at the speed of sound! On the other hand, the proliferation of scientific literature may not be a symptom of ill health but rather a sign of scientific progress *(7)*, since it results from the increasing number of scientists *(8)*:

Year	Number of scientists
1800	1 000
1850	10 000
1900	100 000
1950	1 000 000
1970	3 200 000

Growing numbers of publications also reflect the growth of knowledge. During the whole of 1960 only five publications on prostaglandins appeared, whereas in 1978 five such publications appeared every day. After the discovery of the hybridoma technique in 1975, the number of publications on monoclonal antibodies counted in BIOSIS (Biology and biosciences data base) increased from 10 in 1977 to 28 in 1978, 148 in 1979 and 267 in 1980 *(9)*.

Unfortunately, the flood of publications creates serious problems for the scientific community. The overabundance of information keeps the individual from finding the information he needs; while drowning in information, he is also starving for knowledge.

It is very difficult for people to find the specific information they want. Relevant information is scattered throughout many publications. For example, 54 496 articles on oncology have appeared in 1038 journals *(10)*, 10 286 articles on schistosomiasis in 1738 journals, and 2978 articles on mast cells in 587 journals *(5)*. In the year 2000, the knowledge of 1950 will have doubled, but it will be hidden in 30 times as many publications *(11)*.

Access to all the literature becomes more and more difficult. Libraries are not able to collect all new publications, in part because of rising prices. In the core list of essential journals drawn up by Brandon and updated regularly in the professional journals of medical librarians, the average cost per medical journal was US $11.81 in 1963 and US $59.67 in 1983 *(12)*.

Even if the users get the documents they want, they then face such problems as the language barrier. About 60% of medical publications are issued in English and 9–11% in Russian. The rest are in French or German. An even higher proportion of articles are written in English in some new fields of medical science. Analysing computer searches in MEDLINE, Pfaff *(13)* found that 57.1% of papers on surgery were written in English, 10.7% in German, 7.8% in Russian and 7.5% in French. Of papers on monoclonal antibodies, 95.1% appeared in English.

Scientists in many countries have accepted English as the lingua franca of medicine. One disadvantage of this is the ignorance on the part of American and English scientists of literature not in English.

Terminology, the terms used in certain disciplines or by groups of scientists, raises another barrier to communication. In contrast to that of the new sciences such as nuclear physics, medical terminology, which has developed for many thousands of years, has significant national differences. In addition, the strong relations of medicine to biology, chemistry and physics, as well as to social sciences such as psychology, have enlarged the already unwieldy medical vocabulary.

Since the differentiation of medicine took place not only horizontally, in specialization, but also vertically into the disciplines of basic science, clinical science and medical practice, communication has become more difficult not only between disciplines but also within them. The area most handicapped by this is general medicine which, theoretically, should skim off the cream of scientific progress from all medical specialties for the great subject of concern in medicine: man.

Reading every relevant publication is physically impossible and unnecessary as well, because many publications do not contain any new, useful or important information. Fig. 1 indicates, in an impressionistic way, that the growth of new information is slower than the total growth of information.

Fig. 1. Growth rates of total published information and new information published

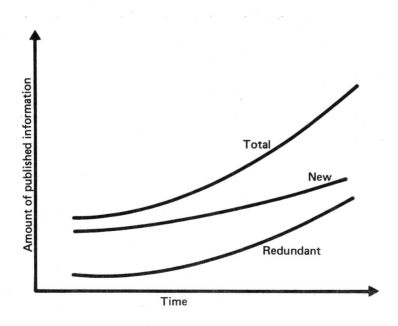

Lebedev *(14)* estimated that 70–80% of all publications are without any practical importance. Warren's results agree *(5)*: of 4000 articles on schistosomiasis only 15% were selected for quality by experts. In other studies experts considered only 13% of 4000 articles on lifesaving therapy of cardiovascular and pulmonary diseases to be essential.

Besides the general fact that scientific work, as a mass phenomenon, has increased the number of not very competent scientists, the main reason for the high proportion of low quality publications is the lack of a simple but effective mechanism for evaluating scientific work and scientists. Unfortunately, a scientist forced to publish or see his academic career perish values the number of his publications more than their quality. Also, original contributions are valued more than surveys. This motivates scientists to use one scientific result for many publications, passing them off as originals by changing titles and arrangement of authors, and to publish preliminary results without verifying them.

The poor quality of scientific work, especially the inappropriate use of statistics, makes a critical selection of publications even more necessary. For example, many reports have shown that about half of all published papers contain statistical errors *(15)*.

The information explosion is therefore mainly the accumulation of paper, the amount of which doubles every 15 years. The growth rates of important new findings are lower *(16)*, as the amount of important knowledge seems to double every 45 years *(17)*.

The problems of quantity and of quality have a negative result: at least 50% of the published literature is never used. A study at the British Library for Science and Technology showed that, in a one-year period, 4800 journals out of 9120 were not consulted; 80% of loan requests were filled from 900 titles and 50% from 40 titles *(18)*. In the Central Scientific Library of the Ukrainian Academy of Sciences, 75% of 2000 journals were not requested during one year, and 8% of the journals filled 80% of the requests *(17)*. In a large medical library with 3000 journals, half of the circulation was accounted for by only 76 titles (2.5%), and only 371 journals (12.4%) were circulated 876 times in a one-month period *(5)*. In a Norwegian dental library with 185 periodicals, 12.9% of the loan requests were filled by 2 journals and 50.1% by 12 journals *(19)*.

The non-use of existing knowledge has several consequences; for example it leads to duplication of work. In the United States, US $2000 million are lost annually because information already published is not known. More than one third of patent applications are rejected because the invention already exists *(20)*. Also, as a result of the effort necessary to find relevant information and weed out the irrelevant, the user loses time both in the search and for creative work.

The difficulties in selecting important information from the mass of publications are particularly great for physicians in medical practice. Needing to keep up with pertinent scientific developments, the physician finds himself swamped with information that he has little time to assimilate or even to scan. The practising physician therefore does not get the information he needs.

Numerous investigations have shown that important new findings in medicine reach this professional group rather late or not at all. For example, a test with 4500 American physicians showed a lack of knowledge on modern antibiotics *(21)*. In another study, 40% of examined physicians did not know any contraindications of oral contraceptive agents, 30% knew one, and 20% knew two *(22)*. Stross & Harlan *(23)* found that only 38 of 137 family physicians (28%) and 42 of 91 internists (46%) were aware of the results of a cooperative trial of photocoagulation in diabetic retinopathy published 18 months before. Only 33% of 229 respondents who were asked to manage two patients' problems involving diabetic retinopathy handled both correctly. These gaps in knowledge harm patients, raise the costs of health care and can hurt a nation's economy.

Whether we consider the proliferation of literature as a normal consequence of scientific progress or describe it as a metaphorical "disease", the information explosion must be controlled. Using the disease model, we should first try to understand the physiology of scientific communication before making therapeutic decisions.

Scientific Communication

Scientific information is a product as well as raw material in the cycles of scientific work (Fig. 2) that can be considered as a complex of information processes:

— collecting already existing information;

— collecting primary data from experiments;

— merging both information categories to form new information, which is released to the scientific community and other users for acceptance or rejection.

Fig. 2. Cycles of scientific work

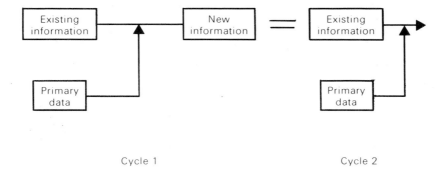

Cycle 1   Cycle 2

The transfer of scientific information from the person who generates it to the person who uses it is called scientific communication (Fig. 3). Although the same people, scientists, act as both generators and users, they prefer the generator's role *(24)*, since publishing serves them better than reading. Incidentally, it would be easier to use scientific information if its generators understood that easy reading is difficult writing. For scientific communication, information travels down two channels:

— informal oral communication by direct contact between transmitter and receiver;

— formal communication using the written word for information dissemination.

Fig. 3. Scientific communication

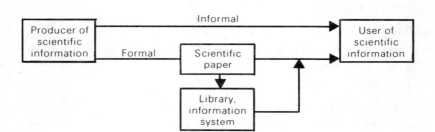

Informal communication

Informal communication, historically the oldest form, has many advantages. It is direct, selective, topical, meets the users' demands, contains know-how and permits response. It is the type of information preferred by the eminent scientists who form the so-called "invisible colleges" and keep each other up to date in this efficient way. In medicine informal contacts with colleagues are often used by clinicians and practitioners.

Informal communication has, however, disadvantages as well. It reaches only a few users, the information cannot be stored and it does not protect the priority of new findings. Scientific meetings constitute an organized form of communication. Their advantages become effective, however, only with small symposia or similar events, and not with congresses assembling thousands of participants, with many lectures and slides, and no time for discussion.

As we shall see later on, certain possibilities of modern technology favour this kind of communication.

Formal communication

Information transfer in formal communication is based on the various forms of scientific literature, of which the scientific paper is still the most important medium. The advantages of this channel include the possibilities of:

— reaching many users;

— storing information;

— protecting the priority of discoveries, an important factor for the motivation of scientists.

It is therefore the most important form of scientific communication. Without the invention of printing by Gutenberg in the fifteenth century, and the introduction of scientific journals in 1665, science would not have progressed as it did. Formal communication continues to be the basis for historical continuity and worldwide cooperation in science.

Formal communication has also produced the information explosion, which is one reason to highlight the disadvantages and failures of this channel.

1.   Its information flows are not selective enough because economic reasons force publishers to aim at a general audience.

2.   The scientific paper very often does not meet the individual needs of users, being redundant for one but lacking necessary details for another.

3.   Feedback is rare.

4.   Information dissemination is delayed because of the time lapse from manuscript submission to publication to perusal.

5.   In most cases scientific papers are not directly transferred to the user, but first acquired and stored in libraries and processed in information systems. Formal communication therefore depends on the efficiency of those libraries and information systems.

Users and their Information Needs in Medicine

The utilization of scientific information is not a passive process. People's information needs regulate it. Information needs are shaped by:

— objective information needs concerning the type of work or problem to be solved;

— subjective or personal information needs determined by the knowledge and experience of the user;

— the ability of the user to recognize his needs, and to express and formulate them either in natural language or, if computer information systems are to be used, in the command language.

Often, the search statement formulated by the user does not reflect his needs. This led Labin *(25)* to the conclusion that the user knows neither what he wants nor how to ask for it. The user's search for information (Fig. 4) is directed not only by his needs, but also by his experience in handling the sources of scientific information, which he often lacks. Finally, the availability of information influences both the need and the search for it. According to Mooers' Law, for instance, a person tends not to use an information system whenever having the information is more painful or troublesome than lacking it.

Fig. 4. Factors related to information needs and information seeking

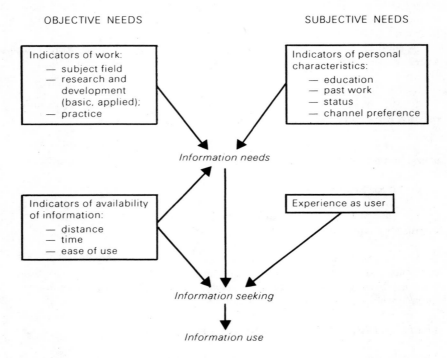

Information needs have several parts:

— the subject matter of the information needed;
— the type of information, such as current information, retrospective searching, and access to primary sources;
— the quality of the information — its completeness, precision and newness.

People doing different kinds of work need different kinds of information.

10

Research workers
Researchers working in basic science, applied research or clinical science are the people who use the most information and seek it most actively. They require highly specific topical information in applied research and thematically broader information in basic science; often they are interested in methodological details. They want access to primary literature. English does not raise a language barrier against them. They use libraries and automated information systems and accept new information technologies. Researchers use existing information systems easily, because these systems are adapted to their needs.

Primary health care workers (practitioners)
This group, although the largest in the medical profession, uses relatively little scientific information. Practitioners have little time or motivation to read. Their continuing medical education aims at keeping them up to date by acquiring new knowledge relevant to their practical work or refreshing their existing knowledge. Secondly, they want to find answers to clinical problems quickly and reliably. They prefer literature in their national language. They want relevant, readable and comprehensible information. Only rarely do they use libraries and information systems in their hitherto existing forms. Oral communication, such as contacts with colleagues and participation in courses, is an important source of information for practitioners.

Health care managers
Scientific information, as opposed to statistical information, is relatively unimportant to health care managers. Top-level managers rely on experts, and those at lower levels say they lack the time to read. They seldom use libraries or information systems.

For managers, information must be not only relevant but also selective, condensed, comprehensible, reliable and practical. Information on trends should be included. This type of complex information should thus combine scientific observations, health statistics and managerial information.

Scientific Literature

The term literature covers a broad spectrum of documentation in print and on computer. There are several types:

— *book*: a non-periodical printed publication of no fewer than 49 pages;

— *pamphlet*: a non-periodical printed publication of no fewer than 5 pages and no more than 48 pages;

— *serial*: a collection of papers without strict periodicity but in numbered issues and with the same title;

— *journal*: a periodical publication with consistent make-up, containing articles, notes, etc.

Serials, journals and newspapers are usually summarized as "periodicals" (see Table 1).

Table 1. Types of scientific documentation

Primary documentation	Secondary documentation
Published / conventional	
Books and pamphlets	
Monographs	Reference literature
Conference proceedings	
Textbooks	
Periodicals	
Serials	Surveys
Journals and magazines	Abstract journals
Newspapers	Bibliographies, indexes
Special types of technical publication	
Standards	
Patents	Indexes
Technical catalogues	Bulletins
Unpublished / non-conventional	
Scientific and technical reports	Library catalogues
Dissertations, theses	Bibliographic files
Translations	
Conference materials	
Official documents	
Descriptions of research projects	

Documents can also be classified by the kind of information they contain. Primary documents record the immediate results of scientific research. Secondary documents are analyses or syntheses of the scientific information contained in primary documents; they give information on information *(26)*.

Different types of document are useful in different stages of scientific work and their use forms a pattern of information dissemination and transfer:

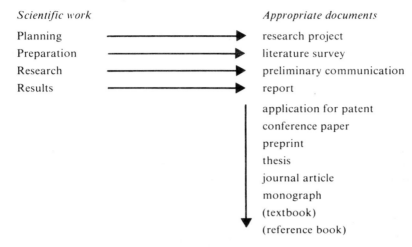

Scientific work	Appropriate documents
Planning	research project
Preparation	literature survey
Research	preliminary communication
Results	report
	application for patent
	conference paper
	preprint
	thesis
	journal article
	monograph
	(textbook)
	(reference book)

Important information sources in medicine

Journals
Today, journals are the most important information source in medicine. About 80% of scientific information passes through this channel. For this reason, most automated information systems store and retrieve information from journals, which in turn has increased the importance of the latter. The journal is useful because it helps scientific information to reach many people relatively quickly.

Journals can be divided by subject into the following groups:

— general scientific journals, such as *Science* and *Nature*;

— general medical journals, such as *Lancet* and *New England journal of medicine*;

— specialty journals, such as *Radiology*;

— subspecialty journals, such as *Neuroradiology*;

— specific topic journals, such as *Atherosclerosis*.

Medical journals can also be classified by their intended readership: researchers, clinical specialists, general practitioners or hospital administrators. Some journals include material interesting mainly to national or local readers, such as *British medical journal* and *Nouvelle presse médicale*. A recent development has been the increasing popularity of medical newspapers such as *World medicine, Health herald* and *Quotidien du médecin*, which provide easily assimilable information culled from other journals, meeting reports and interviews.

This variety of journals, and the original articles, surveys, abstracts, letters, technical reports and book reviews that they present, provides broad but at the same time specific information. The journal allows the reader to browse and keep up to date, as well as to search for specific information. Articles from journals can also be disseminated as copies or as reprints.

Many journals, not only those of professional societies, are social institutions that provide space for communication, exchange of experiences, argument, criticism, speculation and comment, and for promoting medical education in general. But the journal also has its disadvantages.

There are too many journals. The broad supply becomes an excessive supply. Since journals must appeal to a broad audience, information on particular topics is scattered among many journals. The dissemination of relevant articles in many journals follows Bradford's Law of Scattering *(26)* that for each subject a core group of journals can be identified in which these articles appear more often. For instance, 48 of 1038 journals contained 23% of all oncological articles in one series *(10)*; similarly, 19 of 1738 journals covered 33% of all articles on schistosomiasis, and 78 of 587 titles covered 50% of all articles on mast cells *(5)*. These patterns of distribution should influence the acquisition policies of libraries.

In many journals only a small number of articles is relevant to the reader or, as Rossmassler *(27)* states, the journal system "does a good job of assembling knowledge into packages which are about 90% mismatched to the need of users". Many journals are therefore more useful for reference than as general reading.

Journal standards on the style and quality of articles are inconsistent. Many journals are not topical enough. Since most of the medical journals are directed at and read by scientists, they do not meet the specific needs of primary health workers with appropriate contents and style. Up to now the scientific journal has changed very little, but it is developing in some new directions.

The number of medical journals continues to grow. The new titles are mostly specialized and thus reflect the continuing differentiation of medical science. Also, medical newspapers such as *Medical tribune*, *Medical world news* and *Hospital practice* have become popular because they provide easily digested information taken from regular journals, presentations at meetings, interviews, etc.

In 1973 Elsevier launched its International Research Communication System (IRCS) Medical Science, an integrated family of journals in print and as electronic data bases offering rapid publication in less than 30 days and selective dissemination of research data. IRCS uses short papers of approximately 1000 words, which are distributed in the *Library compendium* of all papers published each month, in 32 specialist journals, in 8 special information services and, in cases of general interest, in 3 key journals. Since 1983 IRCS has been available on-line and even provided the possibility for prompt communication between author and reader (see p. 21)

In the USSR, at the All-Union Research Institute for Medical and Medicotechnical Information (VNIIMI) in Moscow, the depot system continues to be successful. Following the Bernal Plan, only abstracts of manuscripts are published, and from these the reader may request a complete copy. This system does not replace the journals, but is an effective addition to them.

The handling of journals has improved: computer systems cover most of the important journals and allow specific searching. People can also use journals to update their knowledge in two ways. First, they may browse in *Current contents*, a publication that lists the contents pages of several thousand journals within a week of publication, with an index of title words and a list of authors' addresses. They may also scan "significant" journals, i.e. those that are most often quoted. The frequency of citation is calculated by a technique known as citation analysis *(28)*. How far, if at all, could such journals act as quality filters *(29)*?

Books
In the natural sciences books play a minor role as sources of information. Thanks to modern printing processes, specialized monographs have come to resemble periodicals more and more. In contrast to the latter, books are less fully represented in automated information systems and thus more difficult to retrieve and to acquire. However, books will maintain their current importance in the future. They are irreplaceable as a means of training and continuing education and as reference works in medical practice.

Grey literature
This term refers to documents that are issued informally in limited amounts and are not available through normal bookselling channels. They are, therefore, difficult to identify and obtain. (By the way, this is completely impossible with "black literature", which contains confidential research results.) There seems to be a great deal of grey literature. The British Library Lending Division (BLLD) annually acquires up to 200 000 reports, while in the USSR about 150 000 research reports are issued per year *(26)*. Dissertations/theses are another important part of grey literature. There were 30 000 in the USSR in 1975, 34 000 in the United States in 1974/75, and about 8400 in the United Kingdom in 1982 *(30,31)*.

Unfortunately the bibliographic control of grey literature is incomplete, and this also makes it difficult to use. The relative importance of grey literature and published literature as sources of relevant information is much debated *(32)*. Attempts to improve access to grey literature include:

— the data base MSIS NIR for which technical reports and dissertations from the CMEA countries are indexed;

— the System for Information on Grey Literature in Europe (SIGLE) of the European Communities, which will be available on-line;

— the World Transindex issued by the International Translations Centre in Delft, Netherlands;

— access to translations provided by the All-Union Centre for Translations of Scientific and Technical Literature in Moscow;

— control and dissemination of the fugitive literature of health service research by the Health Literature and Library Information Service (HELLIS) network of the WHO Regional Office for South-East Asia.

Other media
At present, other media do not play an important part in medical scientific information. Films and audiovisual materials are mostly used for training and continuing education. In some countries the mass media are used to inform not only the lay public but also physicians.

Secondary documentation
As the amount of primary literature increased, so did the necessity for some means of informing people about it. Indexes, bibliographies, abstracts and reviews enable people to find what they want. Many of these secondary documents, produced in libraries, documentation centres and information centres, are current awareness or manual information retrieval systems of either local or general importance. These appear both in print and on computer. The best known are *Index medicus, Current catalogue* of the National Library of Medicine (NLM), *Excerpta medica, Biological abstracts, Chemical abstracts, Current contents* and *Science citation index* (in English); *Bulletin signalétique* (in French); *Medicinskij referativnij žurnal* and *Referativnij žurnal* (in Russian); and *Zentralblätter und Berichte* (in German) *(33)*.

Medical and Health Libraries

Traditional roles and new ways
In the past, medical libraries served mainly as archives and librarians as custodians of the treasures. This has changed; now, "the modern medical library itself serves as the basic element within the infrastructure of local, regional and national medical information systems, for it is the library to which society usually turns first in seeking information" *(32)*. Indeed, the vast majority of scientific documents are accessible only through libraries.

Document delivery, the process of getting a document to the person who wants it through circulation, loan or photocopy, is still a basic function of libraries. Each library has to build an appropriate collection, a task complicated by the necessary consideration not only of users' needs but also of prices and budgets. To solve this problem, librarians must analyse users' needs and identify core and significant documents. Recommended lists of documents, such as the Brandon list in the United States or the list of recommended journals for regional medical libraries in the German Democratic Republic, are useful for some libraries. Audiovisual material forms an attractive new part of the collections of some medical libraries.

After the collection is assembled, it must be catalogued for use. Library catalogues continue to be an important way to manage documents and stored knowledge. The efficient delivery of documents is a more important problem for librarians than the development of a perfect new classification scheme. Subject indexes can be used to overcome the deficiencies of any classification scheme.

In addition to the general problems posed by the information explosion, libraries must also deal with the rising demands for document delivery that result from the increased use of automated information systems. Computer systems have been developed to support and manage library operations such as circulation control, ordering, processing and cataloguing *(34)*. Up to now computers have not changed the work of most libraries, but in the future microcomputers will do so *(35)*.

The introduction of computerized information retrieval systems has had a great impact on the medical libraries. Although libraries had provided information services to readers in the past, on-line searching has now become the most attractive service, and has incidentally increased the reputation of libraries. Today, because libraries operate most terminals used for searching in biomedical data bases, libraries offer people the widest access to the information system. Some countries have other specialized institutions for information services: the Institut für Wissenschaftsinformation in der Medizin (IWIM) in the German Democratic Republic, Deutsches Institut für Medizinische Dokumentation und Information (DIMDI) in the Federal Republic of Germany, the Medical Information Centre (MIC) in Sweden, Dokumentationsdienst der Schweizerischen Akademie der Medizinischen Wissenschaften (DOKDI) in Switzerland, and VNIIMI in the USSR.

Besides the expanded role of librarians as "information brokers", there have been attempts in the last few years to introduce clinical librarians, who work closely with the members of the clinical team to provide them with the services of the library and information networks. "The librarian has come right out of the library" *(36)*. If this effort is to succeed, the attitudes of both parties must change.

Cooperation and organization
Most medical libraries are part of institutions or organizations, such as universities, medical schools, research institutes and hospitals, that adapt their services to their clientele. On the other hand, libraries must cooperate to give access to their stocks and services on the national and the international scale. In the past, people obtained access through inter-library loans, regional or national catalogues, and union lists of periodicals or books. The hierarchical structure of libraries and the regulations of inter-library loans favoured this method.

However, increased demand for publications — for example, in the United States an estimated 20 million items are requested annually through inter-library loans *(37)* — has made the loan system inconvenient. In most countries an inter-library loan is not only slow but expensive. In the United States, for instance, the lending institution charges a fee, usually some US $5–10, for each loan.

One possible answer is the creation of library networks, within a given geographical area or organization, to provide systematic planning of services, coordinated stock selection, union catalogues, and centralized ordering and cataloguing. The first computer-supported network was the Ohio College Library Center, now known as Online Computer Library Center (OCLC) in which 3200 libraries participate *(38)*. OCLC provides shared cataloguing, an on-line catalogue and an on-line inter-library loan system to its members. Other possibilities to improve document delivery are:

— specialized back-up services in libraries such as the British Library Lending Division, and in information centres such as the Centre national de la Recherche scientifique in France, VINITI in the USSR and the Institute for Scientific Information in the United States;

— on-line ordering through such services as DIMDI, the Electronic Maildrop of SDC, Dialorder of Lockheed, and the Automatic Document Request Service of BLAISE; documents can be ordered from the terminal and are posted to the user.

In Europe some projects for electronic document delivery, such as ARTEMIS, ADONIS and APOLLO (see p. 29) have been planned. None of these projects has come into operation yet, and it is not clear when they will and how much these systems and their services will cost. Of course, the capabilities of electronic communication and the fascinating new possibilities of video disk as a storage medium may change the system of document storage and delivery substantially in the future.

Even if the traditional shape of libraries disappears, the library as point of contact between people and information systems, and the librarian as information consultant, will remain in the decades to come. New information services demand new skills of the people who provide them, and librarians in the future will face competition from new professional groups. In 1969 Garfield *(79)* warned librarians that they would disappear like the dinosaurs if they did not adapt to new developments.

Automated Information Retrieval Systems (AIS)

By the late 1950s, traditional information retrieval systems such as bibliographies and indexes could not effectively manage the increasing volume of biomedical information. A new system was needed, both to store large amounts of data and to retrieve relevant information. Automated information systems for literature documentation were introduced to simplify and accelerate the production of bibliographies and indexes. Thus in 1964, MEDLARS became operational at the American National Library of Medicine as the first important automated medical information system, because the printed volumes of *Index medicus* could not contain the flood of new information. Therefore, all documents of secondary importance were stored in automated information systems. Then followed the direct use of information stored on tape, first for the selective dissemination of information, and later for retrospective searches in batch processing, in which references are grouped by time. During this time many computer centres, such as the MEDLARS centres in the United States and other countries, were set up to process these tapes for their users. Information was disseminated more efficiently by the simultaneous use of several data bases, such as at CAN/SDI in Ottawa and EPOS/VIRA in Stockholm.

Automated information systems were widely used only when people could consult them by telephone; in other words when the systems came on line. For example, MEDLINE came on line in 1971. The next step was the creation of networks of telephone communication, such as TYMNET, TELENET, SCANNET and EURONET. With packet-switching, large amounts of data can now be transferred over great distances by satellite, quickly, reliably and economically. The opportunities offered by telecommunication led to the concentration of existing data bases in large host computers. The larger bases and institutions with host computers include: DIALOG (180 data bases), SDC (67), BRS (65), NLM (37), ESA-IRS (36), DIMDI (32), QUESTEL (30), DATA-STAR (21) and MIC (10) *(39)*.

About 1845 data bases existed in 1983. Of these, 762 were bibliographical, 1083 were factual data bases, and 1150 were accessible on-line *(40)*. Hall & Brown *(41)* have estimated that about 70 million bibliographical references were available for on-line searches in 1981. In October 1983 the National Library of Medicine provided 37 bibliographical and factual data bases with a total of 7 million references.

Over the past ten years the number of data bases and their use have increased considerably. The National Library of Medicine yearbooks give the following information for the United States.

Year	No. of on-line searches	No. of terminals
1972	6 000	
1975	400 000	400
1979	1 000 000	1 500
1982	2 000 000	2 000

Similarly, DIMDI provided 8200 on-line searches in 1975 and 80 000 in 1983.

For several reasons, MEDLINE has the largest worldwide distribution.

1.   MEDLINE is the automated version of *Index medicus*, which can be found in many libraries all over the world, so that librarians and users are familiar with the philosophy underlying this system.

2.   MEDLINE was the first system to appear on the biomedical on-line market, and the MEDLARS centres in several countries ensured its expansion.

3.   MEDLINE is supported by the American Government and therefore is cheaper to use than commercial systems.

4.   MEDLINE has a well balanced profile of about 3000 periodicals covering not only basic research but also clinical medicine, including stomatology and nursing. It therefore appeals to many people.

5. MEDLINE covers a smaller range of important periodicals (3000) than either the 4000 of Excerpta Medica or the 8000 of BIOSIS, so people have a better chance of obtaining source material from MEDLINE.

6. MEDLINE has constantly been improved. By permitting searches with command words from the controlled vocabulary of the thesaurus (MeSH) in combination with natural language, it combines the advantages of both technologies.

Although MEDLINE covers periodicals from roughly 70 countries, with 60% of them in English, it is not primarily an international system but an American system that has spread worldwide. American medical literature is relatively over-represented.

Advantages and limitations of automated information systems

The capabilities of on-line searching make automated information systems particularly attractive. There is both the practical and psychological advantage of getting a quick answer to the search inquiry. It is possible to build up very large data bases and nevertheless receive selective information. The flexibility of on-line searching is advantageous to the user of the system. People may use controlled vocabulary of access terms listed in a thesaurus, with varying degrees of sophistication. In certain bases organized on a hierarchical tree structure, such as MEDLINE, one can identify terms that include all these under a given heading; D EUROPE, for instance, retrieves information relative to all European countries. People may also make searches in natural language, using specific words of free text, or making use of truncated terms including a given set of signs, such as MEDIC$ for all expressions beginning with MEDIC. In one series, these include MEDICAID, MEDICAL, MEDICARE, MEDICATION and MEDICINE.

Furthermore, it is possible to print one or more references corresponding to the type of information sought and use the keywords attached to these references to identify relevant search terms, which can be used for further investigation. Combining the advantages of the interacting search vocabularies with the use of Boolean logic — linking the search terms together with AND, OR or NOT — the search can be progressively tailored to the individual user's needs. There are other advantages to the use of automated information systems. For example, people can get access to many different data bases, as well as on-line library catalogues, from one computer terminal. Also, documents can be ordered on-line from the terminal.

However, present automated information systems have their disadvantages.

First, people cannot get all the documents listed as references from their bibliographical searches. Paperchase, now on trial *(42)*, by which people receive only the literature available in a given library, is a partial solution.

The majority of the existing systems are too sophisticated to be used directly by the person desiring information. Most searches are performed by trained search analysts. Because of this delegation of search function to intermediaries, the systems are not exploited to their fullest capacity unless the interested person is also present at the terminal *(43)*.

"Machine-readable databases are multiplying faster than they can be metabolized by the information community" *(44)*. Many of them overlap, so that simultaneous use leads to duplication of references.

Both host computers and data bases vary in subject coverage, record format, data elements included and vocabulary practice. On-line systems vary with respect to command languages, search features, and output formats. This variability is a serious hindrance, since even trained information brokers find it difficult to be fully conversant with several data bases and on-line systems *(43)*.

Although on-line systems are indispensable for complex searches, and on-line searching is cost-effective compared with manual searching, the on-line systems have not replaced traditional retrieval systems for two reasons. Older literature and other sources than journal articles are not covered by on-line systems. Also, simple manual searches are cheaper to perform and can be done where terminals are not in operation.

Only a small number of people use automated information systems, in spite of their increasing rate of use. Even in the United States, many doctors have never heard of MEDLARS.[a] On-line systems are used mostly in the developed countries and by scientists. This may increase the gap between developed and developing countries, as well as that between medical science and health care.

Up to now, automated information systems for literature and those for providing statistical information have developed separately. Modern technology now allows the creation of national health information systems with both national health statistics and health literature. Problems in setting up such a system are obviously not of a technical but rather of an organizational nature.

Finally, although automated information systems are able to retrieve relevant literature, the computers cannot judge the quality of the retrieved documents. People must still evaluate the references to identify the 10–15% of useful and important information.

Future Trends in Information and Communication

This book will not draw a picture of the information age to come, but will mention only some ideas and concepts that might be important in the future.

Developments begun in the 1970s will continue. Bibliographic automated information systems will increase in number and cover scientific literature, including books and grey literature, relatively completely. Microcomputers will promote the establishment of local data bases and encourage local information processing as well as the automation of library housekeeping

---

[a] **Colaainni, L.A.** Paper presented at the International MEDLARS Workshop, Berne, 25–27 October 1983.

operations. This will lead to integrated information and library systems. The current projects for MEDLARS III *(45)* are prototypes of such systems.

New types of computerized system will become more important. Fact retrieval systems allowing direct access to stored facts and data will complete, and later replace, the present document retrieval systems. Some factual information systems, such as TDB and RTECS, are already used in medicine.

Knowledge bases will become a convenient form of easy access to stored knowledge. The hepatitis knowledge base in the National Library of Medicine can be used on-line. It is hierarchically organized by topic with several levels of detail, and experts select and update the current knowledge on hepatitis to be presented in condensed form *(46)*. Other knowledge bases on peptic ulcers and human genetics are in early stages of development *(45)*.

Expert systems, the first results of artificial intelligence, attempt to transfer specialist knowledge into a programme so that the information can be efficiently used by the computer to solve problems *(47–49)*. Systems such as MYCIN and INTERNIST-I help doctors decide questions of diagnosis and therapy. They aid physicians but will not replace them.

While the amount of information will continue to increase, less information will appear in printed form *(50)*. Electronic publishing will become a reality because of its advantages. It is becoming cheaper and allows high-speed and selective transmission of information. "It is cheaper to send light beams through silicon fibers than wood cellulose across the surface of the Earth. We have more light and sand than trees and petroleum" *(51)*.

The first tests with electronic journals are underway. Since 1983 the IRCS Medical Science, besides its printed version, has been available on-line at BRS, and since 1984 at DIMDI, allowing not only on-line access to the full text but also information retrieval. By linking readers' comments directly to the original article it also facilitates communication between writer and reader. On-line journals will appeal primarily to scientists. For other readers, such as practising physicians, paper journals will keep their value for a long time.

New developments in telecommunication will have a great impact on information dissemination *(52)*. Electronic mail, teleconferencing (communication between individuals with computer-aided information and retrieval, high-speed document delivery, graphic projections, etc.), cable television, teletext (two-way telephone-based system linking computer to television sets), facsimile, satellite communication and other developments will improve informal communication both among scientists and between science and other parts of society.

Optical disk technology includes both storage and retrieval of graphics on optical video disks and the storage of digital information on optical digital disks. This technology will improve on-line systems by complementing on-line information with graphics. Furthermore, owing to its high storage density of about 100 000 pages on both sides of one disk *(45)*, electronic transmission facility and the possibility of conversion in different media, it may fundamentally change the system of document storage and delivery *(53)*.

These technological developments will have a great impact on the dissemination, storage and retrieval of information. Scientific communication will also be electronic communication (Fig. 5).

Fig. 5. Electronic communication

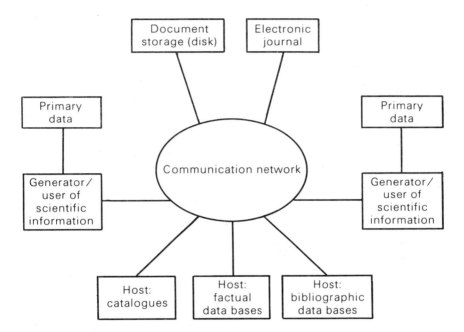

Although technology can change society, "one of the major challenges is to resist 'technological determinism', the tendency to assume that the shape of things to come will be inexorably conditioned by the gathering momentum of technological innovation" *(54)*. Technological development cannot be isolated from economic, political, social and other factors. The development of information and communication in the future therefore depends on their adequate organization. "Can governments", asks Anderla (cited in *54*), "allow automated systems and networks to develop in a chaotic fashion and for strictly commercial motives?".

Computers will not replace human beings as providers of information, although people will perform new tasks in the process. They will manage new technology, extract and evaluate data and information and make syntheses of information. Information professionals with new knowledge and skills may form new professional groups who will produce and provide information.

How independently can people search for information? Vendors of on-line systems have developed special software that facilitates searching by their clients.

— The Knowledge Index of DIALOG/Lockheed offers 16 data bases, including MEDLINE, using 10 commands for home computers.

— BRS/After Dark is a menu-driven home computer search system containing MEDLINE, BIOSIS and HEALTH, in which a person may choose from a menu of programmes.

— BRS/Colleague Medical is a menu-driven system offering to sub-scribers a biomedical bibliographic library including MEDLINE, PRE-Med and HEALTH, and a biomedical complete text library that provides access to the full texts of journals and reference books. For example, the critical care medical library contains the full texts of about 30 major textbooks that cover critical care medicine. The full texts of several important medical journals such as *Lancet* and *New England journal of medicine* will also be available. Especially inno-vative is the BRS plan to make illustrations and graphics available through a video disk attachment.

— BIOSIS has developed B-I-T-S (BIOSIS Information Transfer). Sub-scribers receive the results of SDI profiles on disks or tapes to create their own data bases.

Of course, some people will learn to use computer systems easily. How-ever, before large numbers of people learn how to find the information they need, they must acquire new knowledge and skills to use in the search.

Information for Economy — Economy of Information

The increasing importance of information in modern society is unchal-lenged. The number of people engaged in the generation, collection, storage, retrieval, management, dissemination, evaluation and marketing of infor-mation is growing. According to one study, more than 50% of the American workforce was engaged in information work by 1970 *(54)* and, according to Denison, "about two thirds of the economic growth came about from the increased size and education of the workforce and the greater pool of knowledge available to workers" *(3)*.

Information is a resource with characteristics different from other resources. It is renewable and self-generating, and becomes more rather than less valuable when it is consumed. Furthermore, information is a strategic resource of the developed countries. It is used not only in economic but in political competition. For example, embargo rules keep information from other countries. In addition, information is a source of profit, and in Western countries commercial groups are very much involved in the business of information.

In contrast, the benefits of information are difficult to quantify. For example, Dobrov (55) says: "Very often we cannot exactly define what we get when we receive this or that information. It is only clear that we lose very much not receiving it in time".

The efficient use of information saves other resources. For example, having information such as a scientific result saves the labour of duplicating the experiment. Having information also saves the time that would be lost in the search for it, and the time thus saved can be used for innovative work. Further, information reduces the time span between an invention and its practical application. Weiske (56) reported that 51% of scientists provided with computer-based selective information saved up to 50% of their time through this service; a gain of time was probable, but more difficult to prove, for the other 49%. Dobrov (17) estimates that a saving of half the amount of time at present spent in searching literature would add the equivalent of 100 000 people to the number of scientists in the USSR.

Besides saving other resources, information improves the quality of research, management and health care. The quality of this work and its results depends on the quality of the people involved, and this in turn depends on their education, experience and knowledge.

The importance of adequate information to the quality and costs of health care delivery has been shown in some studies. Scura & Davidoff (57) found that in a random sample of 50 specific case-related literature searches for physicians in a university hospital, including document delivery, patient management was affected in 20% of the cases. This is a large proportion compared with other studies that showed that laboratory tests led to a rate of benefit of only 0.1–5%. The physicians also said that 86% of the literature provided contained new information. In comparison, X-ray examinations were estimated to modify the diagnostic thinking of physicians in emergency rooms 90% of the time. Compared with the costs of X-ray investigation, the total cost of computer searches, librarians' time and photocopying was considerably lower. This finding is confirmed in other evaluations of clinical medical library programmes. Garfield (58) cites a physician: "I found that having the key article is as important as having the lab investigation report". Other studies have shown that new information, perhaps received as part of continuing medical education programmes, improves drug therapy decisions (59,60) and transfusion practice (61), although the impact of continuing medical education cannot always be precisely assessed (62).

The search for and provision of information must be performed efficiently in order to improve the cost–benefit relationship of information. For example, the automation of information and library processes saves labour, time and costs while increasing the quality of the services. Information can also be used efficiently through cooperation and resource sharing.

2

The present situation
in Europe

Special Features of the European Region

In order correctly to evaluate the present situation of health and biomedical information in Europe some special features of the European Region must be mentioned.

1.   In most European countries the libraries and information systems are well developed. Several of these countries have strong national traditions in librarianship, and this can hamper international cooperation.

2.   Europe consists of groups of nations: the industrialized countries of northern and western Europe, with free market economies; the industrialized socialist countries of eastern Europe, with controlled economies; and the less economically advanced countries in the south of the Region.

In addition, groups such as the European Community and the Council for Mutual Economic Assistance (CMEA) have developed their information networks and services in different ways (see Annexes 3 and 4).

3.   Within Europe the existence of more than 20 languages impedes scientific communication. This is one reason for the absence of any internationally significant non-English information system in Europe. Although documents in English currently dominate biomedical literature, there are efforts towards increasing the use of other languages, such as French, and Russian, the working language of CMEA.

4.   Despite the high standard of its scientific and industrial development, Europe is backward in the field of information technology, and especially in its application, compared with the United States. Thus, while the use of on-line systems in the United States rose by 1500% between 1978 and 1982, in Europe utilization rose by no more than 200% *(20)*. Europe depends on the use of American bibliographical biomedical data bases.

Medical Libraries (Document Delivery)

Europe is well provided with medical libraries and expert medical librarianship. Document delivery is generally complete. Although almost all periodicals are secured, acquiring new books and grey literature poses problems. Documents are mostly delivered on a national scale. For example, eastern European literature is difficult for western European countries to obtain. Since no country possesses all literature, copies from the stocks of other countries are accessible through the international interlibrary lending service.

The British Library Lending Division, for example, delivers 18% of its copies to libraries abroad *(63)*. Considerable stocks of medical literature are deposited in the Central Library of Medicine in Cologne, in the State Central Scientific Medical Library in Moscow, in the Library and Information Centre of the Karolinska Institute in Stockholm, in the University Library in Copenhagen, and in the Istituto Superiore di Sanità, Rome. Examples of document delivery centres are the Centre national de la Recherche scientifique and the Institut national de la Santé et de la Recherche (INSERM) in France, and VINITI and VNIIMI in Moscow.

In Europe, medical literature can be ordered on-line through the automated document request service of the British Library Lending Division, from the Medical Information Centre of the Karolinska Institute in Stockholm, and through DIMDI in Cologne. Organized forms of international library cooperation exist among the Scandinavian countries, with the union catalogue of periodicals, and among the CMEA countries with MEDPERIODIK.

The organization of medical library services differs in various countries, because of their different economic development and other factors such as:

— state-promoted information policies in France, the Federal Republic of Germany and the CMEA countries *(63)*;

— central medical libraries in Bulgaria, Czechoslovakia, the Federal Republic of Germany, Hungary, Poland, and the USSR, with similar functions performed by the resource libraries in France;

— regional medical libraries found in the German Democratic Republic and the USSR, partly in the United Kingdom, and planned in France;

— the organization of medical libraries into a network that corresponds to the particular structure of the public health system and is governed by the health ministry, as in all CMEA countries and in the United Kingdom for the National Health Service;

— the development of cooperation among libraries as in the union lists of periodicals used in Italy, Scandinavia, Switzerland and the CMEA countries, and the on-line union lists existing in the Federal Republic of Germany and being developed in France, Sweden and Switzerland.

The efficiency of the medical libraries in particular European countries also varies. The central libraries, the medical libraries of the universities and those in large research institutes are very well equipped. In contrast, libraries in small hospitals are often only poorly developed or not developed at all.

The lack of librarians in these smaller libraries is a serious problem as the physician working at this level gets no help in using the stocks of other libraries through such services as an inter-library lending service. It is mainly in the USSR and other CMEA countries that institutions providing ambulatory health care are equipped with libraries of their own.

The automation of library processes is only beginning. Although the classical medical library still predominates, it is often staffed with librarians who are eager to aid medical staff. It is difficult to assess how active the medical libraries have become. A growing number of medical libraries have become both more active and more respected by installing computer terminals.

In the CMEA countries, active information supply is an important task of the medical information centres that, together with the medical libraries, form an integrated system of scientific information in medicine. Because automated information systems have made documents more accessible, demand for document delivery has risen in Europe in recent years. Economic considerations force the libraries to reorganize their systems of document delivery. The establishment of union lists and cooperation between libraries exemplify the trend towards resource sharing. Libraries must also cooperate in acquiring new literature and in creating the best and most useful collections of literature. The central libraries or resource libraries will perform the important auxiliary service of providing copies of literature that exists only in a certain country in a few copies. Ambitious plans are being hatched for electronic document delivery, through such systems as ARTEMIS, ADONIS and APOLLO, but these have yet to appear in Europe's medical libraries.

The following important health-related data bases are available on host computers based in Europe or easily reached from Europe:

Data base	Host computer
MEDLARS/MEDLINE	DIMDI (Federal Republic of Germany), DATA-STAR (Switzerland), MIC (Sweden), NLM (directly or through BLAISE-link, UK), DIALOG & BRS (USA)
EMBASE	DIMDI, DATA-STAR, DIALOG
BIOSIS	DIMDI, DATA-STAR, ESA-IRS (Italy), BRS, SDC, DIALOG
PASCAL	Télésystème QUESTEL (France), ESA-IRS
ISI	DIMDI
CANCERLIT	DIMDI, MIC, DATA-STAR, NLM
CANCERNET	QUESTEL
TOXLINE	DIMDI, MIC, NLM
HEALTH	DIMDI, MIC, NLM
HECLINET	DIMDI
RESHUS	QUESTEL
BIOETHICSLINE	MIC, NLM
BIRD	G-CAM (France)

These automated information systems are used through terminals installed in medical libraries and information centres, such as IMA in France, DIMDI in the Federal Republic of Germany, DOKDI in Switzerland, or terminals of commercial information brokers. It may be estimated that at least 2000 terminals are being used to find biomedical information in Europe. Most searches are carried out by intermediaries such as librarians, information specialists, biologists and physicians, and not by the person who wants the information. MIC offers an opportunity to these people — mainly physicians in hospitals — to make searches at night, from 7 p.m. to 7 a.m. The programme is called "MEDLINE by night". Access to the various hosts does not pose any technical problem. However, a person making a search must deal both with the varying costs and the varying command languages of the systems. The systems based in the European Community are easier to consult because they share a common command language.

At present, American bibliographic data bases are most widely used in medicine. The large European automated information systems Excerpta Medica and PASCAL are not competitors for the time being. Nevertheless, Excerpta Medica is important in providing drug information, and PASCAL covers important French literature. Also, several European data bases have recently become available on-line: PSYNDEX, HECLINET and ABDA at DIMDI; CANCERNET at QUESTEL; and BIRD at G-CAM. In addition, SWEMED, PRIMLINE and TEDAB are being tested at MIC. On-line use is planned for the data bases of the Department of Health and Social Security in the United Kingdom. European automated information systems functioning off-line include the Soviet systems ASSISTENT and OASNMI, and MEDIK of the CMEA system MEDINFORM. Some countries have small off-line automated information systems that cover a selected theme or themes and are of national significance only. As a whole, the medical literature of Europe is less completely covered by automated information systems than that of the United States. In part, this is because the large European automated information systems aim either at the American market (Excerpta Medica) or at a national market only (PASCAL). American data bases do not always meet the needs of the European public health systems in certain fields. One example of this discrepancy is the data base HEALTH. The European medical literature is covered systematically only in the automated information systems MEDIK and PSYNDEX. MEDIK covers the periodicals of CMEA countries, and PSYNDEX supplements PSYCINFO with periodicals in German.

The creation of a comprehensive new automated information system to compete with existing systems is not a reasonable proposal at present. A higher degree of representation for the European literature in the American systems is desirable, but the development of European on-line systems for certain subjects would be a better solution to the problem. A first rewarding goal might be a European data base on public health. It should include periodicals, health-related grey literature and current health service research projects.

Traditional literature information
Conventional literature information is still highly important to many Europeans. They use printed publications such as *Current contents, Index medicus,*

Excerpta medica, Referativnij žurnal, Medicinskij referativnij žurnal (MRŽ), Bulletin signalétique, and the *Zentralblätter* published by Springer Verlag. Several of these bibliographies or abstract journals appeal to their readers because they are written in their national languages. Such secondary information sources of national, regional or local importance exist in many countries. Information specialists, including physicians in the USSR and other socialist countries, provide non-automated information delivery. Such people synthesize the contents of the literature, not only for surveys, but also to aid special groups of people such as managers and primary health care workers.

Users of Biomedical Information

Research workers
Research workers can find the information they need if they work at medical universities or large research institutes, where they have access to primary literature such as periodicals and to automated information systems. Quantitative differences are due to the different levels of development of the countries in Europe.

Primary health care workers
These people are essential to the achievement of "Health for all by the year 2000". At present they do not get the information they need even though they may be showered with numerous publications such as those from the pharmaceutical industry. Current library and information systems do not provide the kind of information needed by primary health care workers. Therefore these systems are little used, especially as these people are not familiar with them. Studies in several European countries have shown that primary health care workers regularly scan only 3–6 national periodicals. Compared with scientists, primary health care workers do not consume much scientific literature (Fig. 6).

However, contacts with colleagues and participation in scientific events, especially on a local level, are very important sources of information. In the USSR and the United Kingdom, particular emphasis is placed on information for this group of physicians. The findings of several studies have led to the following conclusions on information for primary health care workers.

1. Continuing medical education is very important to the quality of medical care, and therefore cannot be left to the individual physician.

2. Primary health care workers need scientific literature tailored to their particular needs. They must receive the knowledge they want in a comprehensible form.

3. Since primary health care workers do not find their way to the library, librarians must bring the library to them.

Fig. 6. The inverse relation between use of scientific information and responsibility for health care by different categories of physician

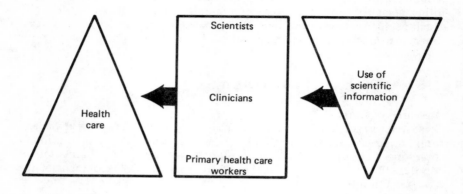

4. Continuing education is important for this group of physicians. Again, knowledge must be transmitted in a form appropriate for the person receiving it. Efforts in this direction are being undertaken in France, the German Democratic Republic, the Federal Republic of Germany, Switzerland and other countries.

5. Primary health care workers need contact with their colleagues. The gap existing between ambulatory and hospital care must be bridged. Activities such as the regular group visits to continuing medical education clinics in the German Democratic Republic provide this professional contact.

Health care managers
The acquisition of scientific information, as opposed to health statistics and management information, is considered to be of minor importance for this group. They use hardly any libraries or automated information systems; these do not answer their specific needs anyway. As yet, no national health information service provides a sufficiently wide range of health-related and biomedical information. Also, such services take the scientific literature too little into account. Good experience of the specific information supply of managers has been gained in the German Democratic Republic, the USSR and the United Kingdom. Information useful in management is also disseminated by IDIS and HECLINET in the Federal Republic of Germany.

Health personnel other than physicians

The information and documentation available to this group,[a] which is an important part of the health care team, are often separate from those available to physicians, as in the libraries of nursing and midwifery schools or in specialist periodicals, and often appear to be much less developed. The importance of regular and specific continuing education for these professional groups, and the need to encourage them to seek and use information, cannot be overemphasized. While physicians have a role to play in these developments, the leaders of these professional groups must take some responsibility for improving information provision and use. The specialized information arising from nursing and related congresses of health care is relevant not only to nurses but to other groups, including physicians, and should be better used.

Other Medical Information Systems

Health information

Health information such as health statistics and literature information are separated in European countries. Medical literature is not included in present national health information systems. Health information systems are relatively well developed in most European countries. Interested readers can refer to other publications *(64–69)*; only a few points will be briefly mentioned here.

Audiovisual materials and films

These have a definite and acknowledged place, particularly in the training of medical students and in the postgraduate education of young physicians. They do not replace but supplement scientific literature. They are also very useful for the health education of the lay public. Their central documentation, in France, the German Democratic Republic, the Federal Republic of Germany and the United Kingdom, avoids duplication of work and facilitates their large-scale application, which because of the language barrier takes place on a national scale. These media should be documented and used in medical libraries.

Mass media

Except for the dissemination of medical information to the lay public, the mass media are very little used for the dissemination of scientific information to the medical profession in Europe. Medico-scientific newspapers exist in France, the Federal Republic of Germany and Italy. Although the *British medical journal* is called a newspaper, it is actually a technical journal.

Until now, little use has been made of television for continuing medical education, except in France and Italy. The use of the domestic television set

---

[a] The limited investigations carried out in the countries visited did not include specific surveys of the documentation and information problems of non-medical health personnel.

for this purpose may possibly increase if teletext systems and home computers deliver specialized information into people's homes.

Drug information
The correct use of drugs is very important in medicine and health care. It also affects the costs of public health systems. In those countries where drugs are an industry, physicians are flooded with large numbers of documents on drugs. In addition to buying a lot of advertising space in scientific publications, the pharmaceutical industry produces an innumerable amount of grey literature and sends its representatives to the physicians. The individual physician cannot cope with this excessive supply. Information retrieval systems without quality filters give him no help.

In the United Kingdom, drug and therapeutic committees and regional drug information centres aid the physician with advice. In France, the Union nationale des Associations de Formation médicale continue (UNAFORMEC), within the framework of continuing medical education, makes critical assessments of drugs independently of the pharmaceutical industry. The measurement of drug consumption is important to health care policy. In Italy, there are plans to measure drug consumption by an automatic reading of the bar code on the drug packages. In the United Kingdom, computers are used to analyse prescription habits in the regions. The timely recognition of adverse reactions is vital to drug safety. In the United Kingdom, physicians are expected to report adverse reactions to drugs voluntarily. However, they have not been quick to do so.

3

The present situation
in selected countries

Bulgaria

Medical libraries
The system of medical libraries in the People's Republic of Bulgaria includes about 100 medical libraries, at the top of which stands the Central Medical Library at the Medical Academy. The most important libraries are found in the 5 medical faculties, the 22 research institutes of the Medical Academy, and the 19 district hospitals. This network contains more than 650 000 volumes and 3467 periodicals, of which the Central Medical Library possesses about 200 000 volumes and 1340 current periodicals.

The Central Medical Library manages and coordinates the work of the decentralized libraries, imports foreign literature and registers the location of the medical books and periodicals in the country. People obtain literature through the inter-library lending service and by ordering copies. The Central Medical Library also collects reports on study trips and congresses, dissertations, WHO literature, and translations.

Further medical literature is available at the Sofia National Library. It also publishes the central catalogue of monographs and periodicals.

Literature information
The use of automated information systems has become more important in recent years. The Central Institute for Scientific and Technical Information in Sofia receives magnetic tapes from large international data bases. The tapes are used for the selective dissemination of information and on-line searches. A network of computer terminals is planned. Important data bases for users in the medical field are:

— BIOSIS, used for about 220 SDI profiles and 400 retrospective searches in 1982;

— INIS, used for 160 SDI profiles and about 20 searches in 1982;

— COMPENDEX, used for 17 SDI profiles and 2 searches in 1982; and

— INSPEC, CIS, AGRIS, CPI, MSIS and NIR.

Searches are done with the help of the MEDINFORM data base MEDIK.

The traditional information processes also supply a great deal of information to scientists and physicians. In addition, these processes overcome the language barrier to a certain degree.

The Centre for Scientific Medical Information (CNIMZ) at the Medical Academy provides information on medicine and public health. It issues:

— general information bulletins containing abstracts from the international literature, surveys and reports for physicians, dentists, pharmacists, and other health workers;

— special information bulletins containing mainly abstracts from the international literature in 18 medical disciplines; and

— surveys as original publications.

The *Abstracts of Bulgarian scientific medical literature* are prepared for foreign users.

The CNIMZ abstracts the international literature reports and other types of document and then supplies this information to senior administrators in the public health service. The Centre publishes abstracts in *Express information for managers*, studies and surveys of health care systems abroad, and detailed information on statistics from these systems. Information is also supplied to managers through such automated systems as:

— the automated information system ESKOM, containing information on study trips abroad and their assessment;

— the AIS HORIZONT, with data on development, programmes, and management operations in developed countries, and 7500 abstracts in Bulgarian, used for selective dissemination of information and searches; and

— the AIS SIRENA, that registers and monitors the planned and realized medical research projects in Bulgaria, and uses the information for selective dissemination of information and searches.

Users of biomedical information
Research workers generally get the information they need. Owing to the language barrier, primary health care workers read little original international literature, but they have access to information on foreign literature through the numerous abstract publications in Bulgarian. These publications are adapted to their needs and are useful both for organized courses and for continuing medical education.

The abstract publications are useful for health care managers, too. The CNIMZ has also developed information services specifically adapted to their needs. Generally, other health workers receive information from other sources, but the CNIMZ publishes a special information bulletin for this professional group, as well. Some physicians can learn to use information systems through lectures, and may be licensed as specialized physicians for medical information and documentation after receiving specific training.

WHO publications are frequently used in the People's Republic of Bulgaria. Literature is deposited in the Central Medical Library, where people may get copies. Furthermore, the WHO literature is regularly indexed and abstracted, and various information bulletins inform their readers about its contents.

Librarians from abroad can be trained at the Central Medical Library at the Medical Academy.

Denmark

Medical libraries
There is no uniform medical library system in Denmark; the University Library, Department 2 (UB2) acts as the central medical library *(70)*. The libraries cooperate only through inter-library lending; other cooperative activities do not exist. New acquisitions of foreign literature are referenced by the Royal Library or the Swedish system LIBRIS. Bio-Med, a union list of periodicals in Scandinavia, is produced by the Library and Information Centre of the Karolinska Institute in Stockholm. The most important medical libraries are the University Library in Copenhagen, the State Library in Aarhus and the University Library in Odense. These libraries cover certain regions of Denmark for on-line searches. There are also medical libraries in hospitals, about 25 of which work full time, though not every hospital has a library of its own. These hospital libraries vary considerably in their efficiency. Owing to the small size of the country, anyone may consult the three large medical libraries. Research institutes and pharmaceutical companies also have well equipped libraries. The National Advisory Council for Danish Research Libraries is a planning, consultative and coordinating organ for research libraries. There is a special group that tries to establish contacts among librarians.

Budget cutbacks, a problem for all libraries, restrict the acquisition of literature and can reduce the number of staff.

University Library, Copenhagen (Scientific and Medical Department)
The library has a stock of about 500 000 volumes, and 8500 periodicals, including 5000–6000 biomedical periodicals. There are also dissertations, a few volumes of grey literature with reports ordered from the BLLD, a small number of audiovisual materials and no microfiches.

Forty per cent of the users of this library come from the University of Copenhagen, and another 40% from other libraries. Eighty per cent of the orders request periodicals. Two thirds of the orders can be handled locally; for the remaining third, other Scandinavian libraries or the BLLD or the Library of Congress are used. About 2500 periodicals are acquired by exchange.

The library has two computer terminals for on-line searches of host computers, such as MIC and DIMDI. MEDLINE is used for 800 searches per year, and Excerpta Medica, BIOSIS, SCI and CAS are used for about 400 searches per year. Some selected dissemination of information (SDI) profiles from EPOS/VIRA and 100 profiles from MEDLARS are also compiled on these terminals. As 90% of the MEDLARS periodicals are available here, people are able to get the periodicals referred to by the computer. This is not easily done with those covered by CANCERLIT or BIOSIS.

Library of the National Board of Health
This library collects literature on public health statistics. It has 27 000 volumes and 330 periodicals, and receives all WHO publications, which are regularly used.
    The following information services are provided:

— circulation of periodicals;

— monthly list of new acquisitions;

— current awareness service with copies from current journals;

— manual searches

— MEDLINE searches (in the University Library, four per month).

Literature information
People search for information in the existing large international information systems, mainly MEDLARS, followed by Excerpta Medica, BIOSIS and others. Terminals, often used by physicians, are installed in the three university libraries and in institutions of the pharmaceutical industry. The Danish terminals are linked with the host systems MIC in Stockholm, DIMDI in Cologne, and sometimes NLM through BLAISE. There is no Danish medical literature information system because the former Index Medicus Danicus has been cancelled. The national bibliography covers only monographs, not journal articles.
    Besides its participation in HECLINET, the Danish Hospital Institute (DSI) has its own data base, with 11 000 references on public health, health economics, hospital management and hospital architecture drawn from 800 journals and 800 books. The literature, 39% of which is in Danish, is indexed with a thesaurus. Interested people can make on-line searches in the DSI data base and in HECLINET on the host DIMDI.

Users of biomedical information
Research workers are the most frequent users of the medical libraries. Their needs can generally be met by existing facilities. Apparently, primary health care workers use libraries and literature systems only to a minor degree. Many of these people seem to restrict themselves to reading certain Danish periodicals. Since continuing medical education is not compulsory, most physicians seem to prefer to seek information from contacts with colleagues and participation in meetings or similar events. Eighty per cent of general practitioners take part in such activities at least once a year.
    Several events and practices seem to indicate improvement in the scientific standard in general medicine and increased motivation to use scientific literature. For example, general medicine has been recognized as an academic discipline, and research on general practice has begun. Local medical

colleges have performed medical audits. The fact that 75% of general practitioners work in group practices is another indication.

The staff of the National Board of Health regularly use scientific literature, particularly in relation to public health issues and statistics.

The libraries of the nursing schools are the most important source of literature for health workers. Nursing literature is also collected in Aarhus.

The language barrier, at least as far as English is concerned, is of minor importance in Denmark. Systematic user training does not exist, and libraries offer no training for foreign librarians.

France

Medical libraries
Medical libraries exist in the universities, hospitals and research institutions, the most important being the Interuniversity Medical Libraries in Paris and Lyon, and that of the Centre national de la Recherche scientifique (CNRS). The microfiche service of the Institut national de la Santé et de la Recherche médicale (INSERM) offers 500 periodicals.

The French libraries have no uniform structure, no hierarchy, and no central medical library. However, the Interuniversity Medical Library in Paris is a resource library for medicine, and that in Lyon serves the same purpose for pharmacy. Plans exist for a regional organization of the medical libraries adapted to the health care structure. A union list of periodicals is being prepared in the DBMIST in Grenoble. On-line requests can be handled. A regional catalogue of this type exists in the Rhône department. The shortage of money is a problem for all libraries.

Library of the Ministry for Social Affairs and National Solidarity
The library is part of the ministry's department of documentation, publications and information and has a stock of 80 000 volumes and 800 current periodicals. Its profile includes general themes of social and health care, statistics, and government documents. WHO literature is included, but little used. Managers make little use of the information provided by the library. The library issues numerous publications such as a selective bibliography, and statistics and bulletins of the Ministry.

Central Medical Library of the Hospitals of Paris
This library is supported by a private "Association for the Development of Documentation in the Hospitals of Paris". It has 20 000 volumes and more than 500 current periodicals at its disposal. Physicians of the Paris hospitals use it most frequently. Copies of documents are made for other people. WHO literature is little used. People may order on-line searches, on MEDLINE at DATA-STAR, PASCAL at Télésystèmes QUESTEL, and, less often, on other data bases such as BIOSIS, and Excerpta Medica.

PASCAL is used to supply French literature. Quick manual searches for abstracts can be made by using the traditional documentation catalogue of the CML. The catalogue has articles from the 100 most important periodicals, classified according to the French classification scheme CANDO.

Library of the Medical Faculty of Lyon
This library contains a pharmaceutical resource library called CADIST with 300 000 volumes and about 900 current periodicals, used by physicians and students. Literature that the library does not possess is acquired by inter-library loan from other libraries of the Rhône department, from France or Switzerland, or from the BLLD. The library has a large collection of dissertations, often consulted. People can learn to do manual searches of their own from videotapes. WHO literature is rarely used. Each year 400–500 on-line searches are made. Eighty per cent are made in MED-LINE on the host system and others in NLM, Excerpta Medica and BIOSIS, or PASCAL on the host system of the European Space Agency Information Retrieval Service (ESA-IRS). PASCAL is used to find infor-mation on French literature or on certain specialties such as psychiatry and anatomy.

Literature information
Access to the large bibliographical data bases is ensured in France. Eighty per cent of the inquiries are answered by MEDLINE. One hundred and seventy-five terminals have on-line connections to the NLM or other hosts such as DIALOG, DATA-STAR and ESA-IRS. The bulk of the searches is made on the data base at INSERM Automated Medical Information (IMA). INSERM is also responsible for training people to make searches. The large French multidisciplinary data base PASCAL which covers 500 000 articles per year (about 40% biomedical literature) and the CANCERNET system are available at QUESTEL. Other French data bases, such as RESHUS, with 3000 documents per year on human sciences of health, have not yet been much used. The Interministerial Mission for Scientific and Technical Information (MIDIST) believes that the existing large bibliographical data bases can satisfy information needs, and that the creation of new data bases to compete with them would not be practical. It is felt, however, that more French literature should be included in these data bases. Furthermore, ways should be found to fill the existing gaps in information. Thus, data bases for public health (as an extension of RESHUS) and tropical medicine are planned. There is also an interesting project to develop a periodicals con-tents list similar to *Current contents* on videotext.

International Children's Centre (ICC), Paris
The International Children's Centre was founded in 1949 and is financed by both the French Government and UNICEF. In addition to education, training and research, the Centre's work includes documentation and information provision. Since 1950, literature on all aspects — medical, social, educational, nutritional — of youth and adolescence has been compiled and indexed. The library has 10 000 volumes and 850 current periodicals, including WHO literature. The evaluation of the literature produces 15 000 references per year, usually with abstracts in English and French. Fifty per cent of the sources are in English, and thirty per cent are in French.

The documentation catalogue contains about half a million references and is used for 300 manual searches annually. There are plans to include associated documentation centres in the developing countries for evaluating literature. In addition to reports and technical reviews the International Children's Centre issues bibliographical bulletins on nutrition, immunization and family planning, as well as the periodical *Courrier* which contains authors' contributions along with a medical, social and public health bibliography. The bibliography is now produced by computer.

The data base of the International Children's Centre (Banque d'Information Robert Debré, BIRD) concentrates on children's problems, including those of developing countries. BIRD also makes use of WHO documents.

The Centre's documentation catalogue has 30 000 references updated each month with 15 000 new references added each year. It can now be searched on-line at the French host G-CAM. Titles, abstracts and descriptions are given in the three working languages, English, French and Spanish. A thesaurus in the three languages is planned for use on-line. The ICC's minicomputer also indexes literature. This information system is attractive not only because of its coverage of a wide range of subjects but also because it provides primary sources.

Interministerial Committee "Audiovisuel Santé", Paris
This institution is a national reference centre for medical audiovisual material such as films, videotapes and slides. Since 1973 it has kept a central file documenting about 5000 audiovisual aids arranged alphabetically, according to authors, special fields and distributors. In addition to technical data on the material, the file provides a short summary, a qualitative evaluation, information on potential users, and the address of the distributor. Interested people may also get title lists on available audiovisual aids. Newly produced material will be evaluated on a fixed scheme in about 30 centres in hospitals. These data form the basis for the central file. Also, slides are produced and collected at the Collège des Médecins for the hospitals of Paris.

Mass media
Up to now the mass media have not been much used to provide information to French physicians. Apart from a television programme for physicians, there was only the journal *Quotidien du médecin* with 40 000 subscribers and a circulation of 57 000. It is directed to all physicians in France, both general practitioners and specialists. In addition to information on professional policy and general issues such as the environment and family planning, it contains medical scientific information from reports on congresses or from foreign medical journals. The authors of the contributions are mostly physicians. The *Quotidien* considers itself a supplement to the specialized professional periodicals.

Users of biomedical information
The information needs of research workers are satisfied in that they have access to bibliographical data bases and to primary sources of information. Primary health care workers apparently make very little use of literature and

libraries although they regularly receive many publications from the pharmaceutical industry. The language barrier is an important factor in this. Medical literature and the present information system do not consider the needs of medical practitioners. MIDIST is planning to investigate these information needs. Contacts among colleagues, including the possibility of obtaining information from hospital specialists, are the most important information sources for these people. A well written doctor's letter, in which a hospital doctor refers a discharged patient back to his own physician, could not only promote communication between hospital and outpatient department but also contribute to continuing medical education, which is voluntary in France. The Union nationale des Associations de Formation médicale continue (UNAFORMEC), a federation of about 800 local and regional associations representing roughly 40 000 physicians working in the outpatient sector, promotes the continuing as well as the obligatory post-graduate education of general practitioners — by holding seminars and courses, by training teachers for local continuing medical education activities, by promoting modern communication methods, and by publishing the journal *Prescrire* exclusively for physicians.

Health care managers, like those of other countries, apparently make very little use of medical literature.

Nurses and other health workers are separately supplied with literature and information. Up to now, this subject has received too little attention, and the information produced for these people is insufficiently used. A MIDIST research project is to investigate this problem. Also, there is hardly any systematic training for people seeking information, although IMA is trying to teach doctors to use automated information systems.

German Democratic Republic

Medical libraries
The medical scientific information system of the German Democratic Republic includes 430 libraries and information centres at universities, research institutes and hospitals. There is no central medical library, although one has been planned. The decentralized institutions are guided and coordinated by the Institute for Scientific Information in Medicine (IWIM). IWIM acts as a central register of library resources. It provides:

— a directory of institutions;

— a directory of bibliographic and abstract information bulletins;

— a union list of biomedical journals;

— a central list of recent acquisitions in a union list of monographs.

In addition, the German State Library in Berlin has a central national catalogue of monographs and periodicals.

IWIM also organizes cooperation between information institutions by such activities as:

— deciding the acquisition policies of the medical libraries;

— planning information activities in accordance with regional and specialized needs;

— setting down standards for structures and processes in libraries and information centres; and

— providing a unified classification scheme for documents.

IWIM also provides continued education for the library staff such as courses on medical terminology, and education for people wishing to use the resources available in the libraries. IWIM also organizes relations with institutions abroad, mainly for cooperation with the socialist countries.

A regional medical library in each of the 15 regions organizes and coordinates the activities of the libraries of its own region. One such activity is the registering of regional medical literature. Specialized libraries and information centres are responsible for certain fields and problems of medicine such as diabetes, oncology and occupational medicine.

The primary literature is supplied in three ways. People may get it from the decentralized libraries directly or through the organized inter-library lending service. They may also get copies or loans of literature from the German State Library, which has a large stock of medical literature. Finally, IWIM can provide articles from 200 periodicals on microfiche.

The medical libraries have a total of about 2300 foreign periodicals. Copies of other foreign periodicals are supplied by the libraries of socialist countries, rather than through the expensive international lending service. IWIM is setting up a new library that will receive about 500 periodicals. Grey literature will also be collected. IWIM stock contains also all WHO publications, reports on study trips and technical reports.

Literature information
People get information in many ways *(71)*; some is provided by computers through on-line searches. Since 1981, IWIM has made 1000 on-line searches every year in the host system, Medical Information Centre (MIC), in Stockholm. MEDLINE is the most popular data base. The State Office for Nuclear Security and Protection against Radiation in Berlin uses the INIS data base in Vienna for the selective dissemination of information and on-line searches. The ASSISTENT data base is used for selective dissemination of information at the Scientific Information Centre of the Academy of Sciences. IWIM also indexes articles in 4000 national medical periodicals per year for the MEDINFORM system. It will be used for the selective dissemination of information and later for on-line searches.

There are computer-based information systems in many fields of medicine, particularly for producing bibliographies and SDI profiles on diabetes mellitus, nutrition, sports medicine, blood donation and transfusion, medical equipment, pharmacy and environmental protection.

Traditional printed bibliographies and abstracts are also used to provide information on occupational medicine, medical laboratory diagnostics, oncology, health education, toxicological chemistry, rheumatology, and others. Such reference publications as *Index medicus* and abstract volumes of *Excerpta medica, Current contents* and *Medicinskij referativnij žurnal* are also used for traditional information activities.

IWIM offers a special publication for the senior administrators of the public health service, *Information for health care managers.* International literature and other information sources are assessed and abstracted. The comprehensive abstracts are written in clear language and make reading of the original source superfluous. The publication also includes studies, documentation, and translations, all of which are adapted to the specific information needs of the managers. Most of this information is distributed selectively.

This management information concentrates on questions of organization and management of the public health system along with developments and trends in medical science and practice. The publication also offers information based on printed data from IWIM, particularly on medical science and the public health systems of foreign countries.

A data base covering current medical research projects in the German Democratic Republic is being prepared.

Users of biomedical information
Research workers generally get the relevant information and primary sources that they need. Primary health care workers study medical literature during their obligatory postgraduate education. After that period, however, they concentrate on national medical literature because of the language barrier. They also read periodicals written specifically for continuing medical education. Though obligatory, continuing medical education is not controlled. Physicians usually attend courses and clinics for continuing education. These have libraries with relevant information. In general, health care managers do not use much primary literature. *Information for health care managers* provides some necessary information.

Other health workers are separately provided with literature and information that is documented especially for them.

Despite a decree from the Ministry for Higher and Technical Education concerning the education of students, the training and education of the people who use information systems are unsatisfactory. Over the last few years, IWIM has issued teaching materials such as guidelines for medical students and instructions for doctors, and has organized lectures for the continuing education of the medical profession. People in the German Democratic Republic can get postgraduate education in medical scientific information.

Federal Republic of Germany

Medical Libraries
The Federal Republic of Germany has many medical libraries, the most important being the Central Library of Medicine in Cologne. The system of medical libraries is integrated into the national library system. Thus it has no structure of its own and is not centrally run. The Working Group of Medical Libraries furthers cooperation among libraries.

The two types of library have different structures *(72,73)*. The general library system is decentralized. Libraries in universities and hospitals are autonomous. The stocks of hospital libraries differ considerably. Each teaching hospital must have a library. The resources of the decentralized libraries are effectively used through a strictly regulated lending service on the regional, interregional and international levels. The service employs such tools as seven central regional catalogues, and the data bank of periodicals (ZDB) of the Staatsbibliothek Preußischer Kulturbesitz in Berlin (West). The ZDB gives the location of more than 340 000 items in all fields, on microfiche or on-line. The libraries cooperate in the acquisition of literature on very important or special subjects.

On the other hand, specialized libraries have a centralized structure. These libraries, such as the Central Library of Medicine in Cologne, are of increasing importance, particularly for the use of automated information systems. The Senckebergische Bibliothek in Frankfurt am Main, covering biological literature, is another important library. In contrast to the decentralized libraries, the specialized libraries have suffered no budget cuts so far.

Central Library of Medicine (ZBM), Cologne
ZBM has a stock of 600 000 volumes and 6600 current periodicals. The library collects the following types of monographic literature:

— all German medical literature;

— important literature in English;

— standard works in other European languages;

— dissertations;

— reports;

— all WHO literature.

ZBM collects the periodicals most often cited by the automated information systems MEDLARS and Excerpta Medica. In 1983, ZBM was used for 205 163 local loans (2.1% of them not settled) and 269 714 inter-library loans (8.0% of them not settled). The inter-library loans included:

— 160 064 orders through the national lending service provided free of charge;

— 13 528 orders through the international lending service;

— 96 122 direct orders provided for a fee.

ZBM uses the NLM classification scheme. A ZBM-owned terminal is used to perform some 1100 searches annually at DIMDI. The terminal is often used for bibliographical inquiries, too.

Niedersächsische Staats- und Universitätsbibliothek, Göttingen
This library fulfils several functions. It runs the Central Catalogue of Lower Saxony, and contains the catalogues of the Central University Library and the library of the Academy of Sciences. The catalogues are available on microfiche or on-line.

Recent medical literature is kept in the Departmental Library of Medicine in 120 000 volumes and 1100 current periodicals. In addition, some medical literature (118 000 volumes and 1073 current periodicals) are kept outside the departmental library and not administered by the library staff, because it is still separately acquired. Audiovisual material and microfiches are not often used to provide information.

The Departmental Library of Medicine makes on-line searches at DIMDI. In 1982 there were 1091 searches; 9% were made by professors, 44% by scientific staff, 38% by students and 9% by other people. The most frequently used system is MEDLARS, followed by Excerpta Medica and BIOSIS.

Gesamthochschulbibliothek, Essen
This modern library has a central library office and five specialized libraries. The Specialized Library of Medicine is housed in the University Clinic and stocks 1200 current medical periodicals. The central office acquires literature and catalogues it on microfiche. WHO literature and dissertations are seldom used. In the Specialized Library of Medicine about 300 on-line searches are made each year at DIMDI, some 40% for people who do not belong to the clinic.

Literature information
According to the Government's information and documentation programme, science information in the Federal Republic of Germany has been organized in specialized information systems. Specialized Information System I includes medicine, biology, social medicine, sports medicine, oncology, and veterinary medicine. The specialized information centre is DIMDI, in Cologne. It was founded in 1969 and became accessible on-line in 1974. Each sector has further information centres. DIMDI now has 32 data bases and has thus become the largest biomedical host system in the countries of the European Community. In 1983 some 80 000 searches were made on-line, 20% more than in 1982. Ten per cent were done at DIMDI itself. The MEDLINE data base is used most. Sixty per cent of the users come from the Federal Republic of Germany and use its several hundred terminals.

The specialized information system tries to integrate the different kinds of information activities by using a uniform operating technology for all computer systems: the software GRIPS, developed and operated at DIMDI. Thus PSYNDEX, which scans and evaluates 150 periodicals in German-language countries, supplements PSYCINFO, a larger system. A similar supplement is planned for BIOSIS.

The following are other important biomedical information systems in the Federal Republic of Germany.

HECLINET
The data base HECLINET provides information on the literature of public health, health care and hospital management. Several institutions developed this system: the German Hospital Institute (DKI) in Düsseldorf, the Institute for Hospital Construction (IFK) in Berlin (West), DSI in Copenhagen,

ÖBIG in Vienna, SKI in Aarau, SPRI in Stockholm, and CMW in Warsaw. About 400 periodicals and other literature are indexed, including WHO literature and architecture and economics periodicals. The clinical literature indexed for MEDLARS is not included in this system.

Each year some 4500 articles are indexed. The participating institutions, mainly DKI and IFK, contribute articles; those in English and German are accepted, and those in other languages are translated into German. Each article is indexed according to terms used in the thesaurus *Hospital care*, which has 1100 descriptors and 3000 related terms. The thesaurus will also be published in English and French. Thirty per cent of the indexed articles are abstracted, and some of these are in English. All the indexed articles are collected and put on magnetic tape at IFK.

The information collected in the HECLINET system is used in several ways. Some is published bimonthly in *Informationsdienst Krankenhauswesen*. The HECLINET data base is used for computer searches. In 1982, 1240 searches were made in the computer in Düsseldorf and Berlin (West). The 55 000 references stored since 1969 are now available for on-line searches at DIMDI. The cooperating institutions in Aarau and Copenhagen, however, receive HECLINET on magnetic tapes to use in their own computers. HECLINET is also used for document delivery. Every indexed article is available on microfiche to the cooperating institutions. In principle, all indexed documents are available.

Institute of Documentation and Information on Social Medicine and Public Health Services (IDIS), Bielefeld

Every year IDIS scans, indexes or abstracts 20 000 articles from 800 periodicals, as well as 1500 references from monographs, WHO publications, and grey literature, to provide information on social medicine, occupational medicine and public health services. The bibliographical description of each article in the catalogue is given in its original language.

The catalogue has its own thesaurus of indexing terms in German, with 3800 descriptors and 2500 related terms. From six to twelve descriptors are assigned to each article. About 50% of the documents in the catalogue are abstracted. The authors of the articles write the abstracts themselves. Forty-five per cent of the abstracts are written in German, 50% in English and 5% in French.

The data stored on magnetic tape are transmitted onto microfiches for the IDIS-MICRODOC catalogue. This printed catalogue is used for manual searches. A system of rotated chains of index terms such as KWOC (Keywords Out of Content) in which keywords appear in different places and forms in the title, combined with main descriptors, permits the linking of several search terms. For the future, the IDIS data base will be available at the DIMDI host computer.

Part of this bibliographic data base may now be obtained as IDIS-SOMED-A at IDIS. The basic store, completed in 1983, refers to 33 000 publications from the years 1978–1982 on occupational medicine and related disciplines. Since 1984 some 5500 references are added annually to update the data base.

The IDIS system also provides the following abstract publications:

— *Dokumentation Arbeitsmedizin* [Documentation in occupational health], with about 2000 abstracts on occupational medicine per year;

— *Dokumentation Gefährdung durch Alkohol, Rauchen, Drogen, Arzneimittel*, with 800 abstracts on addiction problems per year;

— *Dokumentation Impfschäden – Impferfolge*, with about 200 abstracts on vaccination problems per year;

— *Dokumentation Medizin im Umweltschutz*, with about 800 abstracts on environmental hygiene per year; and

— *Dokumentation Sozialmedizin, öffentlicher Gesundheitsdienst, Arbeitsmedizin*, with about 1600 abstracts on social medicine, public health care and occupational medicine per year.

In addition, IDIS publishes irregularly information on special topics. The IDIS information system also provides copies of all referenced primary sources.

CANCERNET, German Cancer Research Centre (DKFZ), Heidelberg
The CANCERNET information system was established in 1969 by DKFZ in cooperation with the French Institut Gustave Roussy. Up to 1976 it was called SABIR-C. The new name underlines the international character of the data base, since oncological centres in Hungary, Italy, Japan, Poland and Yugoslavia have joined the system. Each participating institution indexes its respective national oncological literature for the data base. At present, CANCERNET has 180 000 references, 70% of which are in English. Each year 12 000 articles from 1100 biomedical periodicals are added; 5% of the input originates from books and dissertations. Of the indexed articles, 43% come from periodicals in the United States, 12% from France, 11% from the Federal Republic of Germany, and 7% from the United Kingdom. The thesaurus of index terms is written in English, French and German. It has 5700 main terms and 15 000 subordinate terms. Recently the thesaurus has also been published in other languages. The participating countries receive the data base on magnetic tape. CANCERNET is also available for on-line searches at Télésystèmes QUESTEL in Paris. The German Cancer Research Centre conducts on-line searches on its own computer, although CANCERNET tapes may be included in the DIMDI host system. Other data bases in DIMDI are also used for on-line searches. In 1982, 1182 computer searches were performed, 320 of them in MEDLINE at the DIMDI host, 161 in CANCERNET and 126 in CANCERLIT at DIMDI.

The Springer abstract system
The Springer publishing house publishes abstract journals, for the most important clinical disciplines. Springer issues about 100 000 abstracts each year from about 2000 periodicals. Each volume contains author and subject indexes in German. Although in the past the abstracts were exclusively in German, more and more are now published in English.

Users of biomedical information

In general, research workers use the existing information systems to find the information they need. As in other countries, primary health care workers use the literature, libraries and automated information systems much less. Although, according to recent studies, literature is an important source of information for continuing medical education, workers outside academic circles read specialized publications in German because of the language barrier.

While continuing medical education is considered a professional duty, it is neither obligatory nor controlled. The medical professional organizations offer continuing education activities such as courses, scientific meetings and congresses. These organizations want to improve continuing medical education by improving teaching methods. Other media such as audiovisual aids, films and video disks are of minor importance. The Bundesärzte-kammer, the national association of physicians, has a catalogue of medical films. No information could be obtained on the information needs of health care managers. However, the information services of the IDIS and of the German Hospital Institute are to a large extent adapted to their needs. As a special service, the German Hospital Institute publishes a monthly list of contents pages of health care management journals. Nurses are separately provided with literature. A systematic users' education does not exist.

Italy

Medical libraries

In Italy, medical libraries exist at the universities, at research institutes and, in a very different form, in hospitals. Each institution determines its own policy of document acquisition. There is neither a uniform structure, nor any hierarchy, nor a central medical library.

Two important libraries are the library of the Istituto Superiore di Sanità (ISS) and that of the Catholic University, both in Rome. The most important cooperative activity is the Central Catalogue for Periodicals covering all fields, in which 1500 libraries — among them 300 medical libraries — participate. The catalogue is now available both on paper and on microfiche. The inter-library lending service has no formal rules. The Association of Medical Librarians, formed in 1982, promotes contact among libraries.

The libraries have problems resulting from shortage of money and poor organization.

Library of the ISS, Rome

The library has more than 140 000 volumes and 3500 current periodicals, with little clinical information. It also has a complete collection of WHO literature that is frequently used. Copies are made for external users. An on-line catalogue using the data bases DOBIS and LIBRIS is being prepared.

The ISS houses the MEDLARS reference centre for Italy. About 4000 on-line searches and 400 SDI profiles were made in 1983. MEDLINE and other data bases such as CAS, BIOSIS and PASCAL are used by direct access. Document delivery for MEDLINE citations poses no particular difficulties, as 80% of the periodicals are available in the ISS.

Literature information
Fifty computer terminals in Italy have a direct connection with the NLM. Apparently, the terminals in the pharmaceutical industry use European hosts other than DIMDI. A general overview could not be obtained. A national medical information system does not exist.

Users of biomedical information
On the whole, research workers at universities and larger institutes have access to bibliographical references and primary literature. Primary health care workers use the scientific literature very infrequently, and owing to the language barrier they usually read only Italian periodicals. Continuing medical education in Italy is obligatory, but participation is not controlled. The most widely used forms are courses and meetings. The pharmaceutical industry plays an active role, and experiments are being made with educational television programmes on regional networks.

The supply of scientific literature to health care managers seems to be of no great importance. Managers at the lower levels complain about shortage of time, while those at the top levels consult experts for information.

The information supply to the other health workers is apparently of minor importance.

A systematic users' education does not exist.

Switzerland

Medical libraries
Switzerland is well provided with medical libraries. There are about 300 medical libraries in the universities, the pharmaceutical industry and in hospitals, which can offer postgraduate education only when their corresponding libraries meet certain standards. WHO headquarters in Geneva also has an important library. In the system of public libraries, the Swiss National Library in Berne functions as a national library, containing a bibliography of the national literature and a central catalogue of foreign monographs. Every canton has a cantonal library acting as a depository library of cantonal literature and a focal point of the intercantonal lending service. In contrast, there is neither a hierarchical system of medical libraries nor a central medical library.

Although copies of documents may be ordered directly from any library, the inter-library lending service is based on five regional biomedical libraries. An important means for using the available literature is BIOMED, a union list of biomedical periodicals, compiled by the Commission for Biomedical Libraries of the Department of the Interior. The second edition, published in 1983, records 12 000 biomedical periodicals in 300 Swiss libraries. This system is based on the reports of the participating libraries to the University Library in Lausanne, where the data are stored in a computer. On-line requests can be made. An up-to-date microfiche version of BIOMED is issued every six months. The university libraries voluntarily coordinate their acquisitions of periodicals. The Association of Swiss Librarians, Medical Libraries Section, gives technical advice. Medical literature unavailable in Switzerland is procured from the Federal Republic of Germany or from the BLLD. Medical libraries in Switzerland, too, must apply austerity measures. A general problem is the provision of reports and congress materials.

Literature information

The Documentation Service of the Swiss Academy of Medical Sciences (DOKDI) in Berne is vital in using medical information systems. DOKDI was formerly exclusively connected with the NLM, but since 1982 DATA-STAR has been used for 80% of searches, and the NLM or European hosts for the remaining 20%. In 1983 DOKDI and its branch offices in Geneva and Zurich made 7000 searches, 62% on MEDLINE and 11% on Excerpta Medica, and 350 SDI profiles using a DOKDI-owned microcomputer. Although DOKDI used to have a monopoly on computer services in Switzerland, today there are about 20 terminals in medical libraries and in the pharmaceutical industry. DOKDI still trains people to search NLM data bases. Research workers and hospital physicians use these services most; practitioners use them hardly at all. National biomedical data bases do not exist.

Users of biomedical information

The information needs of research workers are satisfied on the whole. Primary health care workers, however, make little use of medical literature. Continuing medical education is voluntary, but the hospitals and regional medical professional associations organize a large variety of educational events. However, there is neither any national planning of themes nor any coordination. Besides the professional associations the medical faculties of the universities take an active part in continuing medical education. The pharmaceutical industry and the army, which regularly calls up every physician, also provide continuing education, and the Swiss Medical Federation tries to improve teaching methods.

No details were received about the information behaviour of managers. Hospital managers may profit by the educational courses of VESKA and an information service provided by the Swiss Hospital Institute.

Non-medical health personnel are supplied with information separately from physicians. Also, nurses may take part in the annual congresses held by professional societies.

Union of Soviet Socialist Republics

Medical libraries

About 4500 medical libraries and 400 information centres make up the Soviet system of medical and scientific information. The All-Union Scientific Institute for Medical and Medico-technical Information (VNIIMI) coordinates the hierarchical structure of this integrated system along the lines of geographic location and professional specialty. The Central Medical Scientific State Library (GCNMB) governs the activities of libraries. Fig. 7 shows a simplified outline of the structure of the information system.

Fig. 7. The structure of the medical information system in the USSR

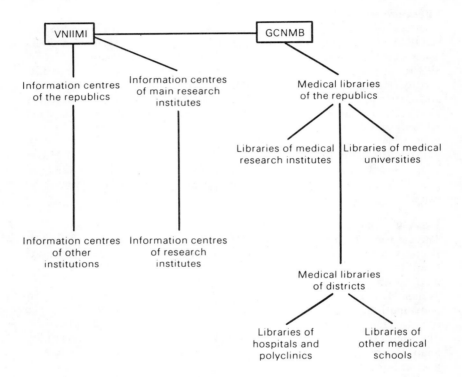

The GCNMB, with over 2 million volumes and about 2000 current periodicals, is one of the world's largest medical libraries. Its stock includes dissertations, technical reports and WHO literature. The library has alphabetical, subject and systematic catalogues. It takes part in computer-based union lists of foreign periodicals and foreign books. The library's collection is used either locally, by more than 55 000 readers, or through the inter-library lending service. Document delivery in the GCNMB is about 1 700 000 units a year, including copies. People or institutions that subscribe to contents list bulletins can request copies of articles mentioned in the bulletins from VNIIMI. Copies may also be ordered by telex.

Documents provided by the All-Union Institute for Scientific and Technical Information (VINITI) are important for medical research, since they give researchers access to the primary sources that are only abstracted in the *Referativnij žurnal (RŽ)*.

The GCNMB provides extensive information services:

— publication of current monthly bibliographic cards in 41 series, numbering about 2 million cards a year;

— publication of current and retrospective special bibliographies, and lists of recent acquisitions such as *New books on medicine*, and *Literature for the practising physician* with annotated recommendations;

— 400 manual retrospective literature searches per year; and

— about 4500 hours per year of oral translation of foreign articles into Russian in the presence of a user.

Efforts are made in the USSR to manage the grey literature. The medical libraries of the Ukrainian SSR in Kiev and Kharkov, for example, publish registers of conference papers and technical reports of institutes that are not available in bookshops.

A special form of literature provision is the deposit system. A total of 6500 manuscripts, published in the *Medicinskij referativnij žurnal (MRŽ)*, have been deposited in VNIIMI and other information centres, so that people may have access to the complete manuscript.

Literature information
Documentation on medical literature forms part of the National System of Scientific-Technical Information (GSNTI). The system consists of:

— 10 all-union institutes, including:

  VINITI (information in natural sciences and technology),
  VNTICentre (technical reports),
  CNIIPI (patents),
  INION (information in social sciences),
  VCP (translations);

— 86 central branch information centres;

— local information centres, including 109 inter-branch local and 243 branch-related information centres; and

— 11 000 information centres in institutions.

The GSNTI has a central management, applies uniform methods and works on the principle of the coordinated division of labour. Information on foreign medical literature flows down to the people using the decentralized information institutions in several forms, such as bibliographies, abstracts and surveys, after being scanned and indexed in the all-union institutes to avoid duplication of labour. On the other hand, information on the national literature is gathered at the decentralized institutions and aggregated at the all-union institutes. A characteristic feature of the Soviet information system is the high professional qualifications of the staff; 20% of the staff in medical information centres are physicians.

Information services used for the selective dissemination of information are important in the decentralized information institutions. The significance of automated information systems to these services has increased in the last ten years. A network of automated information centres is now being established in the Soviet Union. This includes OASNMI (Automated Branch System of Information in Medicine) on the VNIIMI computer, for which articles in foreign and Soviet periodicals are indexed in VNIIMI, in GCNMB and in large research institutes. OASNMI is used for the selective dissemination of information, while retrospective searches have played a minor role only.

The data bases MEDIK of MEDINFORM and ASSISTENT in VINITI are used in the selective dissemination of information. About 6000 biomedical periodicals are indexed for the biomedical part of ASSISTENT, which covers the following fields: virology, morphology, pathology, physiology, genetics, oncology, immunology, biophysics, molecular biology, pharmacology, toxicology and bionics. Some 75% of the sources are written in English, 14% in Russian. Title words, keywords and classification terms are used in computer searches. The automated information system ITOGI produces surveys in the aforementioned fields for VINITI.

VNIIMI uses the data bases of the International Centre for Scientific-Technical Information in Moscow (Conference Paper Index, Science Citation Index, MSIS NIR) for the selective dissemination of information. The data base INIS, as well as the data bases of DATA-STAR, Excerpta Medica, BIOSIS and PREMED, are used for on-line searches.

VNIIMI provides a great deal of information through the following traditional information services.

1. The bibliography *Medicine abroad* covers 100 000 titles annually in 66 series; these cards are used not only by individuals but also for building up decentralized data bases. VNIIMI uses this retrieval system for about 1200 manual retrospective searches per year.

2. *MRŽ* is an abstract journal in 22 series with a total of over 40 000 abstracts per year. *MRŽ* focuses on clinical medicine and abstracts 16.3% of its articles from periodicals of the USSR, 11.9% from periodicals of socialist countries and 71.8% from periodicals of other countries. Specialists write the highly informative extracts in Russian.

3. *Express information*, a publication issued in 16 series, offers comprehensive abstracts and surveys on clinical medicine. It is intended for medical practitioners.

4. *Obzory* (Reviews) consists of the yearly publication of about 40 extensive surveys written by specialists and reflecting the state of knowledge in various fields.

5. *Register of information materials on medicine and public health* is a monthly publication that records the bibliographies produced in Soviet medical libraries and information centres, translations of medical literature, newly deposited manuscripts, and recent documents explaining methods and setting standards for Soviet public health care.

6. *Register of deposited documents* is a publication covering deposited documents. People also value the current awareness service, the term for the selective distribution of the contents pages of journals, for its usefulness in ordering copies of articles.

The decentralized information centres use both central information services and the results of their own information activities to provide people with bibliographic, abstract and factual information.

Special selective services provide information for the senior staff of the public health service. One such service provided by VNIIMI is DOR (Selected Management Information) which sends abstracts from international periodicals to health service managers in accordance with their individual needs.

Managers receive an annual report on developments in medicine at home and abroad; they can also make individual requests for information. Automated factual information systems can be used for such requests, for example, in registers of current research projects and the results of medical research.

Users of biomedical information
Research workers get all the information they need and the language barrier is of no significance for this group.

Primary health care workers prefer literature written in Russian. In addition to national periodicals and literature published especially for this group, such as monographs and documents explaining methods and setting standards for the public health system, such publications as the abstract journal *MRŽ* and *Express information* provide practitioners with information in Russian on world medical progress.

The GCNMB issues a special bibliography for this group, called *Literature for the practising physician*. Practitioners are required to continue their medical education by participating in compulsory general or thematic courses. The Institute for Postgraduate Medical Education usually organizes these courses. Medical literature is very important for continuing medical education and is actively promoted by the medical libraries. Many public health care institutions regularly hold information days, readers' conferences and similar events.

Other health workers get professional literature from the libraries of nursing schools and from local libraries. These people are also required to continue their education by attending courses or seminars at the institutions where they work; physicians take an active part in these courses.

Educating people to find and use relevant information is a traditional part of medical training and continuing education. The active information propaganda of the libraries and information centres may now be a more important part of this process. Many institutions have physicians, called physician information specialists, who are responsible for the use made of medical literature.

United Kingdom

Medical libraries
The United Kingdom is well equipped with medical libraries, which can be divided into the following main types:

— universities and medical schools;

— royal colleges;

— private societies such as the Royal Society of Medicine;

— hospitals and postgraduate medical centres;

— research institutes such as the National Institute for Medical Research (NIMR);

— government, in the Department of Health and Social Security (DHSS);

— pharmaceutical companies.

First and foremost, every library acts as a part of the institution to which it belongs. There exists neither a national plan for an a uniform system of medical libraries, nor a central medical library. However, the medical libraries can borrow literature they lack from the multidisciplinary British Library Lending Division (BLLD). The BLLD charges a fee for lending any of the 57 000 periodicals in its stock. For certain sources the rich libraries of the Royal Society of Medicine and of the British Medical Association give back-up services for the BLLD. There is no union catalogue for the holdings of all medical libraries. However, the British Library publishes *Serials in the British Library*, which lists its own periodical holdings and those of 17 other important libraries in all fields. There are also regional union lists of holdings in several regions, that promote inter-library lending and coordination. Such cooperation also exists between the libraries of the University of London.

Attempts have been made for several years to organize the libraries of the National Health Service (NHS) according to its regional structure, and some progress has been made in the Oxford region. The Oxford Regional Library System includes:

— the Cairns Library;

— the libraries of the postgraduate centres at the general district hospitals;

— branch libraries at other hospitals;

— libraries of the nursing schools.

However, the medical libraries of the universities are not included in the system.

The regional librarian is subordinate to the Regional Health Authority and is supported by a library committee. His tasks are to advise and support the libraries, to train library staff, to monitor library activities and to organize cooperation within the library system. He must also compile a computerized list of regional periodicals. The list includes, however, only the holdings of the NHS libraries. This list forms the basis for the regional inter-library lending, and 50% of the requests are first satisfied in the region, free of charge. Further, the regional librarian organizes the on-line searches. At present, the Oxford region has four terminals at its disposal. One terminal is to be installed in each district. The NHS pays for the searches, DATA-STAR is most frequently used in searches, and BLAISE is mainly used for the selective dissemination of information.

The Cairns Library functions as a resource library for the Oxford region. No corresponding central regional library exists in other regions. Furthermore, the development of this regional system is still incomplete; at present there are only six full-time regional librarians. The regional librarians cooperate in an NHS regional librarian group. Although it has no central management functions, this group is important to the development of medical librarianship. The Medical, Health and Welfare Libraries Group of the Library Association is also of great significance, publishing among other things a list of medical libraries *(74)*.

Economic pressures encourage effective cooperation among the various libraries.

Library of the DHSS

This consists of a main library and four branches, and has a large stock of 200 000 volumes and 1800 current periodicals. Apart from scientific literature, documents of the DHSS, the NHS and the Government are also collected. Furthermore, it is a depository library for WHO publications. The library not only provides sources but also gives bibliographical information, using BLAISE, DATA-STAR and DIALOG for on-line searches.

The library publishes numerous current awareness bulletins based on the scanning and indexing of the new literature. These include monthly published title lists such as *Current literature on health services, Current literature on general medical practice,* and *Health buildings library bulletin,* or abstract bulletins such as *Hospital abstracts* which publishes 150 abstracts per month, the monthly *Social service abstracts* and the quarterly bulletins *Nursing research abstracts* and *Selected abstracts on occupational diseases.*

Since 1983 the library has had an efficient computer of its own, a PRIME minicomputer, using STATUS software. The library has automated its processes and produces data bases such as Hospital Abstracts and Social Service Abstracts. Since 1985, DHSS data bases have been accessible on-line through hosts in the United Kingdom and in continental Europe (DATASTAR).

Library of the British Medical Association (BMA)
The library has more than 100 000 volumes and 1100 current periodicals, along with pamphlets, reports and WHO publications. Most of the books are acquired without payment because they are review copies for the *British medical journal.* The library is used mainly by members of the BMA, but other libraries also take advantage of it. At present, the catalogue is being organized on the NLM classification scheme, and computerized at the same time. The library also performs 200 information searches annually, 120 of which are automated. DATA-STAR is usually used for on-line searches. Manual searches of *Index medicus* are free of charge.

Charing Cross Hospital Medical School Library
The library has 10 000 volumes, of which 350 are current periodicals, and about 600 items of audiovisual material. It serves 2000 people, 800 of whom are medical students. The catalogue uses the NLM classification system and will be accessible on-line in the near future. People can read in the library or get their own copies of articles. Literature that is not available in the library's own stock is procured mainly from the BLLD. Each month 20–25 on-line searches are carried out, usually in DATA-STAR, plus some 10 manual searches. Library seminars are held for students. There are also courses for secretaries, because the senior staff send their secretaries to the library. Interested people can do searches in Index Medicus and Science Citation Index by themselves. Some WHO literature is available, but it is seldom used. Great value is placed on close contacts with the users. Since the library is open until 9 p.m., it is very convenient for physicians.

Library and Information Centre of the King's Fund Centre
The King's Fund Centre is an independent institution financed by donations. It promotes the development of health care and health service management by research projects, organization of conferences, and other contacts. Its library takes part in these activities. It has a stock of 13 000 reference books and about 300 current periodicals for health care management problems. Librarians scan the incoming literature, and copies of relevant articles are stored in dossiers, classified on a modified BLISS system and by country. This permits quick access to relevant facts and data. These dossiers may only be read in the reading-room. In addition, the library handles written inquiries and telephone requests.

Literature information
Bibliographical information is compiled from NLM data bases such as MEDLARS, as well as those of other large medical automated information systems such as Excerpta Medica and BIOSIS. European hosts, especially DATA-STAR, are also used. BLAISE allows access to information on books from the United Kingdom MARC and the Library of Congress MARC and conference reports from the Conference Paper Index.

National information systems provide hardly any literature information, except for the DHSS data base. The British Council publication *British medicine* is a current awareness service on recent British medical literature.

Users of biomedical information

Research workers can find necessary information through the existing library system and automatic information systems. As in other countries, however, primary health care workers use literature and libraries much less, although some libraries have special services to help them. Postgraduate medical centres have libraries to support continuing medical education, which is voluntary in the United Kingdom. Because of great interest in this problem, the particular features of this group of physicians have been studied. These investigations identified among others the following reasons for their information behaviour: absence of motivation and awareness of information needs, no knowledge of the library system and of the literature, lack of time, and great distance to the library *(75–77)*. Further studies are under way, such as a research project in the Wessex region to investigate the information needs of community medical practitioners.

An improvement of the existing situation requires such changes as:

— development of appropriate forms of literature;
— more active role of libraries;
— user training;
— use of modern technology.

As in other countries, the significance of the literature for health care managers seems to be underestimated, although the information systems of the DHSS and the King's Fund Centre could be adapted for this. The Cambridgeshire Area Information Research Project concludes that medical libraries may play a useful role for the information supply of the NHS district manager *(78)*.

Apparently, literature for other health workers is stored separately from literature for physicians, in libraries of schools of nursing. However, *Nursing research abstracts* is kept in the DHSS Library.

With some exceptions, there is no systematic education for people seeking information.

4

Conclusions and recommendations

Special Features of the European Region

In order to evaluate and improve the availability of biomedical information in Europe some special features of the European Region must be kept in mind. Traditional library practices, political, social and economic conditions, and underdeveloped information technology impede the cooperation between European nations that is necessary for the better provision of information.

Medical Libraries (Document Delivery)

Europe has many medical libraries and expert medical librarianship. Document delivery, particularly of periodicals, is generally complete, although new books and grey literature are more difficult to get. Documents are mostly delivered on a national scale. While no country possesses all literature, the stocks of other countries are accessible through the international network of lending libraries.

The automation of library processes is only beginning. Active information supply is becoming an important task of the medical information centres which, with the medical libraries, form an integrated system of scientific information in medicine. Because of automated information systems, demands on document delivery have risen in Europe in the last few years. As a whole, the trend towards resource-sharing and coordination has grown.

All important international biomedical data bases are available in Europe for on-line searching. Their use has constantly increased over the last few years. At present, it is mainly American bibliographic data bases that are being used in medicine, but over the last few years several smaller European data bases have become available on-line, and Eastern European automated information systems are available off-line. Some countries have small off-line automated information systems of national significance only. As a whole, the medical literature of Europe is less completely covered by automated information systems than that of the United States. The creation of a new, comprehensive automated information system to compete with the existing systems is not a reasonable proposal at present. European on-line systems should, however, be developed for certain subjects, such as public health.

Traditional Literature Information

Conventional literature information is still highly important to many Europeans using biomedical information. Such secondary information sources of national, regional or local importance exist in many countries. Information specialists in the USSR and other countries provide non-automated information. It is thus possible to analyse and evaluate the contents of the literature not only for general surveys, but also for services adapted to the needs of special groups of people, such as managers and primary health care workers.

Users of Biomedical Information

Research workers in most European countries can find the information they need if they work in medical universities or large research institutes, where they have access to primary literature and automated information systems. Quantitative differences are due to the different levels of development of the countries in Europe.

Existing library and information systems do not meet the information needs of primary health care workers, managers and other health workers. Therefore these systems are little used, all the more so as the users are not familiar with them.

User Education

No European country has a sufficiently systematic user education. Only local activities exist, thanks to the initiative of local librarians (particularly in the United Kingdom).

WHO Literature

WHO literature seems to be regularly used in Europe, in different forms and by different people. Scientific and technical WHO publications are used by scientists and experts, and the ministries of public health and other policy-makers use statistical and health policy-related WHO publications. However, although WHO literature is valued in the CMEA Member States it seems to be generally less used in Western European countries. This may be because the distribution of WHO literature within countries is uneven, so that it is not known or easily accessible to interested people. It may also be seen as less relevant to the developed countries of Europe and suffer from a language barrier in some countries.

Training for Librarians

Every country visited is willing to train librarians from abroad to use new information systems.

Recommendations to Member States

1.   Individual countries should increase the responsibility of their public health systems for the development of medical libraries and documentation units, and organize the health literature service as part of the national health information services.

2.   They should improve the literature and information supply to primary health care workers and non-physician health personnel.

3.   They should create specific information services for high-level managerial staff.

4.   They should promote the education of users of information, and their awareness of and willingness to use available resources.

5.   They should improve the quality of identification, storage, use and dissemination of European medical literature.

6.   They should extend the bibliographical control of European medical literature, particularly literature on public health and grey literature.

7.   They should promote the use of WHO publications.

8.   They should support less developed countries by providing services and manpower training.

Recommendation to the Regional Office

The Regional Office for Europe could assist Member States in these activities by emphasizing health literature programmes, promoting training and international professional contact among medical librarians, promoting the education and awareness of users, and publicizing experiences and problems in biomedical information, medical librarianship, and continuing education. Groups working for the improvement of information supply to primary health care workers and health care managers, as well as for the bibliographical control of the European literature on public health and the analysis of the use to which WHO publications are put, could begin these developments.

References

1. *Draft medium-term plan (1984–1989)*, 2nd part. *VII. Information systems and access to knowledge*. Paris, UNESCO, 1982.
2. **Mihajlov, A.I. et al.** *Grundlagen der Informatik*. Berlin, Staatsverlag der DDR, 1970.
3. **Naisbitt, J.** *Megatrends: ten new directions transforming our lives*. London, Macdonald & Co., 1984.
4. News and notes: views. *British medical journal,* **282**: 1879 (1981).
5. **Warren, K.S.** Selective aspects of the biomedical literature. *In:* Warren, K.S., ed. *Coping with the biomedical literature: a primer for the scientist and the clinician*. New York, Praeger, 1981, pp. 17–30.
6. **Mihajlov, A.I. et al.** *Naučnye kommunicacii i informatika*. Moscow, Nauka, 1976.
7. **Goffman, W.** The ecology of the biomedical literature and information retrieval. *In:* Warren, K.S. ed. *Coping with the biomedical literature: a primer for the scientist and the clinician*. New York, Praeger, 1981, pp. 31–46.
8. **Mihajlov, A.I.** [Scientific and technical information and effectiveness of science]. *Rivista dell' informazione,* 3(1): 74–77 (1972).
9. **Kraft, R.-P. et al.** The growth of publications on monoclonal antibodies 1975–1981: a bibliometric evaluation. *Journal of cancer research and clinical oncology,* **105**: 199–201 (1983).
10. **Sandor, L. et al.** [Analysis of the structure of cancer literature based on SABIR-C. III. A survey of the distribution of the world oncological publications from 1969–1974]. *Zeitschrift für Krebsforschung,* **86**: 209–218 (1976).
11. **Dobrov, G.M.** *Wissenschaftswissenschaft*. Berlin, Akademieverlag, 1969.
12. **Kronenfeld, M.R. & Gable, S.H.** Real inflation of journal prices: medical journals, U.S. journals, and Brandon list journals. *Bulletin of the Medical Library Association,* 71(4): 375–379 (1983).
13. **Pfaff, G.** Citation indexes and language. *Lancet,* 2: 1166 (1983).
14. **Lebedev, G.A.** O razvitii sistemy naučno-techniceskoj informacii. *Naučno-technisceskaja informacia,* 1(4): 3–8 (1975).
15. **Glantz, S.A.** Biostatistics: how to detect, correct and prevent errors in the medical literature. *Circulation,* **61**: 1–7 (1980).

16. **Rescher, N.** *Wissenschaftlicher Fortschritt: Eine Studie über die Ökonomie der Forschung.* Berlin and New York, de Gruyter, 1982.
17. **Dobrov, G.M.** *Wissenschaftsorganisation und Effektivität.* Berlin, Akademieverlag, 1971.
18. **Urquart, D.S.** The use of scientific periodicals. *In: International Conference on Scientific Information.* Washington, DC, National Academy of Science, 1958, pp. 471–479.
19. **Riordan, P.J. & Gjerdet, N.R.** The use of periodical literature in a Norwegian dental library. *Bulletin of the Medical Library Association,* **69**(4): 387–391 (1981).
20. **Lamprecht, H.** *Moderne Informations- und Kommunikationstechnologien in den hochentwickelten kapitalistischen Ländern.* Berlin, WIZ der AdW, 1983.
21. ... Antibiotics again. *British medical journal,* **1**: 1107–1108 (1976).
22. **Jacobs, W.** Deutschlands Ärztefortbildung: Überblick, Kritik und Anregungen. *Der deutsche Arzt,* **27**(3): 30–50 (1977).
23. **Stross, J.K. & Harlan, W.R.** The dissemination of new medical information. *Journal of the American Medical Association,* **241**(24): 2622–2624 (1979).
24. **Price, D. de Solla.** *Research on research: journeys in science.* New Mexico, 1967, p. 10.
25. **Labin, E.** Informationsanalyse und Datenbanken. *In: 2. Europ. Kongreß über Dokumentationssysteme und -netze, Luxemburg 27–30 Mai 1975.* München, Verlag Dokumentation, 1976.
26. **Mihajlov, A.I. & Giljarevskij, R.S.** *An introductory course on informatics/documentation.* Paris, UNESCO (UNESCO COM/WS/147).
27. **Rossmassler, S.A.** Scientific literature in policy decision making. *Journal of chemical documentation,* **10**(3): 163–167 (1970).
28. **Garfield, E.** Significant journals in science. *Nature,* **264**: 609–615 (1976).
29. **Lock, S.** Information overload: solution by quality? *British medical journal,* **284**: 1289–1290 (1982).
30. **Koppitz, H.-J.** Ungehobene Schätze in unseren Bibliotheken. *In: Jung, R. & Kaegbein, P., ed. Dissertationen in Wissenschaft und Bibliotheken.* München, Saur, 1979, pp. 29–39.
31. **Vickers, S.** Sources of access to theses. *Interlending and document supply,* **11**(4): 140–144 (1983).
32. **Cummings, M.M.** Health science libraries: infrastructure for information services. *In: Health information for a developing world. Fourth International Congress on Medical Librarianship, Belgrade, 2–5 September 1980.* Belgrade, Postgraduate Medical Institute, 1980, Vol. 4, pp. 5–17.
33. **Morton, L.T., ed.** *Use of medical literature,* 2nd ed. London, Butterworths, 1977.
34. **Grefsheim, S.F. et al.** Automation of internal library operations in academic health sciences libraries: a state of art report. *Bulletin of the Medical Library Association,* **70**(2): 191–200 (1982).
35. **Rowat, M.J.** Microcomputers in libraries and information departments. *Aslib proceedings,* **34**(1): 26–37 (1982).

36. **Carmel, M.** Beyond networking. *In: Health information for a developing world. Fourth International Congress on Medical Librarianship, Belgrade, 2–5 September 1980.* Belgrade, Postgraduate Medical Institute, 1980, Vol. 4, pp. 107–119.
37. **Garfield, E.** While you're up, dial me an OATS — we are still waiting for the document delivery revolution. *Current contents,* **10**(50): 5–10 (1982).
38. **Haas, W.J.** Computing in documentation and scholarly research. *Science,* **215**: 857–861 (1982).
39. **Forster, A.** External databases: an overview. *Aslib proceedings,* **35**: 346–353 (1983).
40. *EUSIDIC database guide 1983.* Oxford, Learned Information, 1983.
41. **Hall, J.L. & Brown, M.J.** *Online bibliographical databases,* 2nd ed. London, Aslib, 1981, p. 213.
42. **Horowitz, G.L. & Bleich, H.L.** Paperchase: a computer program to search the medical literature. *New England journal of medicine,* **305**(16): 924–930 (1981).
43. **Doszkocs, T.E. et al.** Automated information retrieval in science and technology. *Science,* **208**: 25–30 (1980).
44. **Gechman, M.C.** Machine-readable bibliographic data bases. *In: Annual review of information science and technology,* 7: 323–378 (1972).
45. **Cummings, M.M.** The National Library of Medicine. *In:* Warren, K.S., ed. *Coping with the biomedical literature: a primer for the scientist and the clinician.* New York, Praeger, 1981, pp. 161–181.
46. **Bernstein, L.M. et al.** The hepatitis knowledge base: a prototype information transfer system. *Annals of internal medicine,* **93**: 169–181 (1980).
47. **Duda, R.O. & Shortliffe, E.H.** Expert systems research. *Science,* **220**(4594): 261–268 (1983).
48. **Garfield, E.** Artificial intelligence: using computers to think about thinking. Part 1. Representing knowledge. *Current contents,* **11**(49): 5–13 (1983).
49. **Garfield, E.** Artificial intelligence: using computers to think about thinking. Part 2. Some practical applications of AI. *Current contents,* **11**(52): 5–17 (1983).
50. **Pool, I. de S.** Tracking the flow of information. *Science,* **221**(4611): 609–613 (1983).
51. **Aveney, B.** Electronic publishing and the information transfer process. *Special libraries,* **74**: 338–344 (1983).
52. **Raitt, D.I.** Recent developments in telecommunications and their impact on information services. *Aslib proceedings,* **34**(1): 54–76 (1982).
53. **Goldstein, C.M.** Optical disk technology and information. *Science,* **215**(4534): 862–868 (1982).
54. **Cronin, B.** Post-industrial society: some manpower issues for the library/information profession. *Journal of information science,* 7: 1–14 (1983).
55. **Dobrov, G.M.** Beschleunigung des wissenschaftlich-technischen Fortschritts durch bessere Informationen. *Informatik,* **21**: 8–11 (1974).
56. **Weiske, C.** Kosten von Magnetbanddiensten. *Nachrichten für Dokumentation,* **24**(3): 97–101 (1973).

57. **Scura, G. & Davidoff, F.** Case-related use of the medical literature: clinical librarian services for improving patient care. *Journal of the American Medical Association,* **245**(1): 50–52 (1981).

58. **Garfield, E.** The impact of hospital libraries on the quality and cost of health care delivery. *Current contents,* **11**(8): 5–10 (1983).

59. **Johnson, M.W. et al.** The impact of an educational program on gentamicin use in a teaching hospital. *American journal of medicine,* **73**(1): 9–14 (1982).

60. **Avorn, J. & Soumerai, S.B.** Improving drug-therapy decisions through educational outreach: a randomized controlled trial of academically based "detailing". *New England journal of medicine,* **308**(24): 1457–1463 (1983).

61. **Handley, S.** Does continuing medical education affect health care: a study of improved transfusion practices. *Minnesota medicine,* **66**: 167–180 (1983).

62. **Melmon, K.L. & Blaschke, T.F.** The undereducated physician's therapeutic decisions. *New England journal of medicine,* **308**(24): 1473–1474 (1983).

63. **Busowietz, M.** Aspekte der Entwicklung im System der Informations- und Literaturversorgung in Skandinavien, Frankreich, Großbritannien und den USA. *Nachrichten für Dokumentation,* **33**(4/5): 178–188 (1982).

64. **McLachlan, G., ed.** *Information systems for health services.* Copenhagen, WHO Regional Office for Europe, 1980 (Public Health in Europe, No. 13).

65. **Strickland-Hodge, B. & Jeqson, M.H.** Usage of information sources by general practitioners. *Journal of the Royal Society of Medicine,* **73**: 857–862 (1980).

66. **NHS/DHSS Health Services Information Steering Group.** *Converting data into information: proposals formulated by members of two workshops held in March 1982 about the management arrangements required for collecting valid clinical data and providing a district information service.* London, King's Fund, 1982.

67. **Körner, E. & Mason, A.** A national approach to health service management information services: the work of the English health services information group. *Effective health care,* **1**(1): 59–65 (1983).

68. *VESKA annual report 1982.* Aarau, Veska, 1983.

69. **Fernandez Perez de Talens, A. et al., ed.** *Health information systems: the Italian approach.* Amsterdam, IFIP-IMIA Fourth World Congress on Medical Informatics, 1983.

70. **Kajberg, L.** Libraries and librarianship in Denmark. *IFLA journal,* **5**(2): 78–90 (1979).

71. **Institut für Wissenschaftsinformation in der Medizin.** Medizinische Informationsmittel aus sozialistischen Ländern. *DDR-MEDIZIN-Report,* **12**(8): 675–730 (1983).

72. **Deutsche Forschungsgemeinschaft.** *Überregionale Literaturversorgung von Wissenschaft und Forschung in der Bundesrepublik Deutschland: Denkschrift.* Boppard, Harald Boldt Verlag, 1975.

73. **Kraft, R.P.** *Analyse und Darstellung des funktionellen Ablaufs der Beschaffung von Primärliteratur bei Bibliotheken nach einer Recherche in bibliographischen Datenbasen des In- und Auslandes.* Heidelberg, Gesellschaft für Information und Dokumentation, 1981 (BMFT-FB-ID 81-003).

74. *Directory of medical and health care libraries in the United Kingdom and Republic of Ireland,* 5th ed. London, Library Association, 1982.

75. **Ford, G. et al.** *The use of medical literature: a preliminary survey.* Wetherby, British Library, 1980 (British Library Research and Development Report 5518).

76. **Cockerill, P.E.** *Information and the practice of medicine: report of the medical information review panel.* Wetherby, British Library, 1981 (British Library Research and Development Report 5605).

77. **Gann, R.** *Help for health: the needs of health care practitioners for information about organizations in support of health care.* Southampton, Wessex Regional Library and Information Service, 1981 (British Library Research and Development Report 5613).

78. **Morgan, P.** The Cambridgeshire area information research project. *MHWLG newsletter,* No. 20: 12–26 (1983).

79. **Garfield, E.** Citation indexing: historio-bibliography and the sociology of science. *In*: Ellison-Davis, K. & Sweeney, W.D., ed. *Proceedings of the IIIrd International Congress of Medical Librarians, Amsterdam, 3–9 May 1969.* Amsterdam, Excerpta Medica, 1970, pp. 187–204.

World Health Organization

Health Literature Services

The main objective of the Health Literature Services is to secure the availability of scientific, technical and managerial health and health-related information for the WHO Member States. Some of the special tasks of the service are:

— developing and strengthening the health literature services in Member States;

— establishing regional networks to promote cooperation and resource sharing;

— fostering information transfer on important health matters between countries;

— improving human resources through the training of library staff and of people using information services; and

— providing support to developing countries with bibliographical information and primary literature.

The programme emphasizes the education and training of personnel in libraries and information centres, because the quality and efficiency of the health literature services depend essentially on the staff's qualifications. In the developing countries, the development of management techniques and skills and attitudes of library cooperation is particularly important. In the developed countries as well, librarians must enlarge their knowledge of the handling of modern technology and automated information systems and the application of international standards. They must learn to see themselves as active parts of the health care team.

The service also promotes cooperation between libraries on national and regional levels. Resource sharing is of vital importance, especially in the developing countries. An important means of cooperation is the documentation of existing resources, such as union lists. Five libraries in the Eastern Mediterranean Region have compiled a union list of publications, and seven medical libraries in the African Region have done the same. The South-East

Asian Region has developed an important means of cooperation: the HELLIS (Health Literature and Library Information Service) system was begun in 1979. The highest development has been achieved in the Region of the Americas with the regional centre for information, BIREME.

The service promotes bibliographic control of biomedical and health-related periodical literature not covered by the existing information systems. Such information can be collected in a Regional Index Medicus. Indexes such as this have been created in two regions with Index Medicus Latino-Americano and Index Medicus for South-East Asia, and are being prepared in the African and the Eastern Mediterranean Regions.

Grey literature, which is not covered in the present information systems but which may contain important information, is also to be brought under bibliographic control, to be disseminated after critical assessment. A project for the collection, bibliographic control and dissemination of grey literature was launched by the Member States of the South-East Asian Region in 1983. A similar project is in preparation in the Western Pacific Region. WHO headquarters participates in such activities by providing guidelines on methods and through *WHODOC: Index to WHO technical documents*. *WHODOC* is a bimonthly publication of WHO headquarters that lists WHO documents of general interest from WHO headquarters and regional offices. The titles of the documents, with indications of location, language, and with index terms mostly taken from MeSH, are given in the order of WHO programme areas. About 1000 documents will be listed each year. In this manual form *WHODOC* is a current awareness service rather than a tool for retrospective searches.

The service provides direct support to developing countries in their use of automated information systems, such as MEDLINE, PASCAL and others, and by providing copies of periodical articles. Apart from providing services of its own WHO also tries to recruit institutions to make MED-LARS searches and provide back-up photocopy services. Corresponding services are rendered by Australia for the Western Pacific Region, by Sweden for the South-East Asian Region and by Italy for several African countries.

The service perceives the development of national infrastructures of information services as the way to solve the problems of cooperation. Apart from organizational aid, the most important task is to develop an awareness within the senior administrators of the public health system that a national policy for strengthening the medical libraries and information system is necessary. Also, ministries of public health must feel responsible for the development of the health literature system. The establishment of national information systems is an essential precondition for effective international cooperation. This can be done if people fully appreciate the importance of library and information services to health. This means, among other things, that the medical librarian must be seen as a full member of the health team. Also, the current isolation of the various health information systems must be ended. National health information systems must be viewed as coordinated complexes of management information, health statistics, and health literature, that satisfy the information needs of different types of people.[a] When this is done, information can be spread better and further through international cooperation.

WHO headquarters and the regional offices must put the service into practice. In addition to designing and planning, headquarters is already directly involved in providing services, consultants, training, standardization and a health literature services programme newsletter. WHO has also established a core list of health and biomedical periodicals and tested the applicability of microcomputers in medical libraries.

The health literature services of WHO also include the headquarters library, an important medical library with a considerable stock of 2500 current periodicals, 40 000 volumes and more than 250 000 documents and publications from WHO, the United Nations and Member States. The library offers such services as the circulation of periodicals for the staff, a current awareness room and loans and copies of literature for headquarters and Regional Office staff and other libraries. About 33 000 copies are provided each month, including 300 copies of articles for developing countries per month. The library also provides the staff with literature from other libraries such as BLLD. A list of recent acquisitions and the list of the serials in the WHO headquarters library give additional information. The library also provides about 100 SDI profiles and retrospective searches on computer systems; MEDLINE is used most frequently. About 60 searches are made per month for staff and 90–100 for developing countries. Bibliographical and factual information is provided on request, along with WHODOC. A microcomputer was installed in 1986.

The WHO health literature services promote and develop health literature services in the developing countries in particular, where they have serious shortages of literature, technology, qualified personnel and modern information systems.

Europe has been mentioned very little at the sessions of the Advisory Committee on Medical Research Subcommittee for Information. Because of the rather good medical library system in most European countries, regional health literature services have not yet been developed, apart from the provision of computer searches for certain countries.[b]

WHO Publications

WHO publications from headquarters, regional offices and the International Agency for Research on Cancer form an important part of the world's biomedical literature.[c] All WHO publications are sent free of charge

---

[a] *National health information system: guiding principles.* Geneva, WHO, 1980 (document NHIS/80.1 Rev.1).

[b] *The WHO health literature services programme.* Geneva, WHO, 1983 (unpublished document).

[c] **Rhee, H. & Sicat, F.C.** *The publications of the World Health Organization: their storage, accessibility and retrieval in small libraries.* Geneva, WHO, 1983 (document HLT/83.3).

to ministries of health or national health administrations and to the designated WHO depository libraries in each country. Selected publications are also sent free of charge to medical institutions, health centres and experts according to a mailing list indicating their relevant subjects. WHO publications can also be obtained from WHO headquarters or through booksellers designated by WHO in almost all Member States.

Unfortunately there is neither any clear information on how these publications are used in Europe nor much feedback from readers.

The following attempt to describe and assess the use of WHO literature in Europe is therefore based on opinions gathered from readers and librarians whom the author met on his visits to several countries.

The good news is that WHO literature is regularly used in Europe. Scientists and experts use scientific and technical publications. Ministries of health and analogous institutions use publications on statistics and health policy. WHO publications are also used in information systems on public health such as DHSS, IDIS and HECLINET.

There is, however, a general feeling that WHO literature is used less fully than it should be, that many publications do not reach the readers they are intended for and that readers do not fully understand them. Publications from the Regional Office for Europe are even less known than those of headquarters.

Of course, WHO publications share the problems of other literature. For example, each piece of literature is relevant only for a definite group of people. Also, primary health care workers and health care managers do not read very much.

WHO literature is not fully used for several reasons. For example, readers often do not know about WHO publications or how to get them. Many people do not know about the existence of relevant WHO publications. Catalogues and bibliographies inform librarians, not managers and primary health care workers. In such countries as the German Democratic Republic and Switzerland, however, recent WHO publications are regularly announced in journals for physicians, who can then use this information to order what they want. WHO literature is insufficiently represented in existing on-line information systems. Publications from the Regional Office for Europe are hardly included at all. As yet, there is no other way to do retrospective searches for WHO literature with on-line technology. Scanning WHO publications directly takes too much time. Also the publications are not available everywhere. People often have difficulty in finding the publications they want. The series publications cover many different topics, and books on one topic can appear in different series.

WHO literature is sometimes hard to get. Some librarians even consider it as grey literature. In most countries, except most CMEA countries, WHO literature is not systematically collected but distributed at random. Depository libraries very often act as archives rather than provide back-up services and copies. Paradoxically, in some western countries the use of the book trade for the dissemination of WHO publications is made more difficult by the fact that they are too cheap, while in other countries the number of copies distributed free of charge is insufficient, because additional copies must be paid for in hard currencies.

The foreign language barrier keeps literature from readers who do not know the official WHO languages, especially English. The primary health care workers are most handicapped by this.

The style of WHO publications is sometimes criticized for being too general or too non-committal, the language of an organization that has to consider the interests of all its Member States.

Also, some people say that WHO literature is less relevant to the developed countries of Europe. This suggestion, however, cannot apply to the publications of the Regional Office for Europe.

Apart from the necessity of regular reader feedback, the best ways of improving the use of WHO literature are to eliminate its character as a marginal type of scientific literature, and to promote its effective use in the ways used to promote scientific literature in general. For example, current awareness mechanisms should be established. Classified lists of titles or more convenient abstracts of new publications should be published in national medical journals and/or as a part of a widely distributed WHO publication or service. When they have this information, people will be able to order the items they want. Also, an automated retrieval system for WHO publications and documents should be established. It would facilitate retrospective on-line searches as well as the selective dissemination of information. In addition, this system would have positive psychological consequences: on-line searches would not only be effective and comfortable but status symbols as well. Such a non-commercial data base might facilitate the necessary introduction of modern information technology in some countries.

Finally, the availability of WHO publications should be improved by using the system of medical libraries. The depository libraries should provide back-up services, and many medical libraries, mainly those of regional significance, should collect WHO literature.

WHO and its Member States must undertake these actions. The Member States should be encouraged to provide translations, abstracts and reviews of WHO literature for their people.

WHO Documents

In headquarters and the Regional Offices, technical documents are produced in small numbers, usually only in certain languages or for a restricted list of recipients, as a communication medium for staff, experts and collaborating institutions. These documents have the character of internal working documents, but they often contain important information that is also useful for people outside WHO. It is sometimes claimed that it is exactly these documents that contain essential facts. *WHODOC* now allows these people to retrieve and use a limited selection of such documents. However, *WHODOC* seems to be relatively unknown in the European Region.

International Agency for Research on Cancer (IARC), Lyon
The International Agency for Research on Cancer (IARC) generates and disseminates information that is useful for the primary prevention of cancer.

IARC has developed programmes to identify the causal factors in human cancer and the individuals or population groups who risk developing cancer.[a]

IARC gets most of its information from two sources. The first is scientific literature. The IARC library has 200 current periodicals and access to oncological data bases. In 1982 these data bases were used for 312 on-line searches and 23 SDI profiles. Scientific experts also contribute information. The Agency subjects all information to critical analysis and evaluation, transforming data into useful information.

IARC makes a major contribution to biomedical information with its series of IARC Monographs on the Evaluation of the Carcinogenic Risk of Chemicals to Humans. The aim of the Monographs is to identify potential carcinogenic risks due to exposure to chemicals or complex mixtures that occur in the environment, and to assemble and evaluate existing knowledge on chemicals known or considered to be potentially carcinogenic for humans. The Monographs are compiled by working groups of experts who consider all the published data relevant to the assessment of the carcinogenic risk of the chemicals under discussion, including data on chemical production, occurrence, experimental carcinogenesis, toxicology, mutagenicity and epidemiology. During a ten-day working period, the experts make a critical evaluation of all available data and prepare a text for publication.

The critical evaluation of all available data, leading to an evaluation of the evidence of carcinogenicity, is intended to assist national, public and occupational health authorities in making decisions on preventive measures through the control of exposure. By 1984, 32 Monographs covering more than 680 chemicals and complex mixtures have been published: 7 industrial processes and 23 chemicals or groups of chemicals have been identified as being causally associated with human cancer, while 14 others were evaluated as probably causally related to human cancer.

The Agency also periodically publishes an Information Bulletin on the Survey of Chemicals Being Tested for Carcinogenicity. Information is collected by a postal survey. The most recent Bulletin, the tenth, gives data from 103 institutes and 16 different countries on 1043 chemicals.

IARC Scientific Publications, at present numbering 55, include the proceedings of meetings, textbooks on experimental tumour pathology, textbooks on statistical methods in cancer research and a compilation of world cancer statistics, *Cancer incidence in five continents*, published every five years. The average distribution of the Scientific Publications is close to 2500. They go mostly to people and institutions engaged in cancer research in most parts of the world. The distribution of the IARC Monographs is close to 4500, of which a substantial percentage goes direct to government agencies involved in regulation.

Although these publications certainly reach the most eminent oncologists in the world, it is doubtful whether they reach all potential readers. It is not clear what significance this information, important as it is to

---

[a] *Annual report, 1982.* Lyon, IARC, 1983 (document SC/19/2; CC/24/2).

health policies, may have for health care managers. IARC publications have the same problems as other WHO publications.

IARC processes information and supplements traditional information systems by acting as a clearing-house for current research in cancer and epidemiology. About 3000 research workers are written to annually and asked to report on current research projects in the field of cancer epidemiology. Incoming data are checked and processed by a computer at the German Cancer Research Centre in Heidelberg. On the basis of these data the annual *Directory of on-going research in cancer epidemiology* is produced. The data on the research projects are arranged by the countries in which they took place. Comprehensive registers facilitate the selective retrieval of desired information, such as: research workers, key-words, site, chemicals, cancer type, professional category and list of cancer registers. This clearing-house function is part of the ICRDBP: following the publication of the Directory the information is entered into the CANCERPROJ system.

This information on current research projects is more topical than scientific literature and thus promotes timely communication among scientists. The 1983 Directory lists 1302 projects in 64 countries. Unfortunately, not all countries participate fully, so that the Directory can only incompletely reflect the situation in the world.

United Nations Educational, Scientific and Cultural Organization (UNESCO)

With the Intergovernmental Conference for the Establishment of the World Science Information System in 1971, UNESCO began to play a more active role in the worldwide improvement of information services. The UNISIST programme was launched in 1973 with the goal of creating a global network of information systems with the voluntary cooperation of existing and planned national information systems.

The UNISIST programme promotes national infrastructures of information (NATIS) as a precondition for international cooperation. Some results of the scientific and methodological work in this field include guidelines for such structures (1–6).

The UNISIST programme tries to develop and apply norms and standards of information and documentation as a means to connect information systems (7–10). UNISIST also promotes modern technology such as the development of the software package CDS/ISIS (11) to process its own document collection and for use in Member States, including versions for IBM mainframe computers running the DOS and VM operating systems. This software is being used by 79 institutions in 29 countries, by 10 United Nations organizations and 5 other international organizations. A mini/micro version of CDS/ISIS, written in PASCAL, is nearing completion. This will support all the features of the mainframe version of CDS/ISIS and will enable people in Member States to move from a small multi-user system to a large mainframe version with complete file compatibility, at the record and field level, and without the need for retraining.

At present, a software package is being developed for microcomputers at IMD, Graz, Austria. A further system acts as a generalized data base management system, for use in both bibliographical and factual information management. It will improve — mainly in the developing countries — the conditions for launching national automated information systems. The system is now being tested in Nairobi. To assist developing countries in the selection of hardware for libraries and information work, UNESCO supports the International Centre for Information Handling Equipment in Zagreb.

UNISIST trains people to use information systems and to help others do so. It gives seminars and courses but also provides teaching materials and publications *(12-17)*. It organizes aid for developing countries by providing methods, personnel and technology. It has also developed its own specialized information systems such as:

— Science and Technology Policies Information Exchange System (SPINES);
— Development Science Information System (DEVSIS);
— International Information System on Research in Documentation (ISORID); and
— Data Retrieval System for the Social Sciences and Humanities (DARE).

The concept of UNISIST is now integrated into the General Information Program. Therefore several specific programmes were adopted at the General Conference in 1982 for the 1984–1989 period. UNISIST will improve access to information through modern technology, standardization and interconnection of information systems. The objectives of this programme are:

— to develop standards, rules, methods and other tools for the processing and transfer of specialized information and the creation of compatible systems;
— to enable developing countries, individually or on a regional basis, to set up their own data bases and to have access to existing data bases;
— to promote the development of specialized regional information networks; and
— to contribute to the harmonious development of compatible international information systems among the organizations of the United Nations system.

UNISIST will also help to develop infrastructures, policies and training required for the processing and dissemination of specialized information. This programme should help the Member States to set up national information systems, to improve the various components of these systems, such as libraries and information centres, and to train information specialists to instruct and train others in the information and library sciences.

Finally, UNISIST will improve UNESCO information and documentation systems and services. The objectives of this programme are to ensure the harmonious development of the documentary services and information systems of UNESCO; to encourage increased participation by Member States in these systems; and to improve the flow of information and documentation within UNESCO.

Part of these activities is a subprogramme that will place particular emphasis on putting the information produced by UNESCO on computer, on the circulation of material in microfiche form, and the maintenance of the CDS/ISIS-CAN/SDI software packages and their introduction into Member States and international organizations *(18)*.

80

References

1. *UNISIST guidelines on the planning of national scientific and technological information systems.* Paris, UNESCO, 1975 (SC/75/WS/39).
2. **Vilentchuk, L.** *Guidelines on the conduct of a national inventory of scientific and technological information and documentation facilities.* Paris, UNESCO, 1975 (SC/75/WS/28).
3. *Guidelines for the national bibliographic agency and the national bibliography.* Paris, UNESCO, 1979 (PGI/79/WS/18).
4. **UNESCO, IFLA.** *Guidelines for the compilation of union catalogues of serials.* Paris, UNESCO, 1982 (PGI/83/WS/1).
5. **Dulong, A.** *Guidelines on referral centres.* Paris, UNESCO, 1979 (PGI/79/WS/4).
6. **Wollman, P.** *Guidelines on the conduct of a national inventory of current research and development projects.* Paris, UNESCO, 1975 (SC/75/WS/13).
7. **Vajd, E.** *UNISIST guide to standards for information handling.* Paris, UNESCO, 1980.
8. **IFLA International Office for UBC.** *Manual on bibliographic control.* Paris, UNESCO, 1983 (PGI/83/WS/8).
9. **Dierickx, H. & Hopkinson, A.** *Reference manual for machine-readable descriptions of research projects and institutions.* Paris, UNESCO, 1982 (PGI/82/WS/10).
10. *Information transfer*, 2nd ed. Geneva, ISO, 1982 (ISO Standards Handbook 1).
11. **Poncelet, J.** *Guidelines for the establishment and evaluation of services for selective dissemination of information.* Paris, UNESCO, 1980 (PGI/BO/WS/14).
12. **Atherton, P.** *Guidelines for the organization of training courses, workshops and seminars in scientific and technical information and documentation.* Paris, UNESCO, 1975 (SC/75/WS/29).
13. **Lancaster, F.W.** *Guidelines for the evaluation of training courses, workshops and seminars in scientific and technical information and documentation.* Paris, UNESCO, 1975 (SC/75/WS/44).
14. **Saunders, W.L.** *Guidelines for curriculum development in information studies.* Paris, UNESCO, 1978 (PGI/78/WS/27).
15. **Neelameghan, A.** *Guidelines for formulating policy on education, training and development of library and information personnel.* Paris, UNESCO, 1978 (PGI/78/WS/29).
16. **Grolier, E.** *Register of education and training activities in librarianship, information science and archives.* Paris, UNESCO, 1982.
17. **Atherton, P.** *Handbook for information systems and services.* Paris, UNESCO, 1977.
18. *Draft medium-term plan (1984–1989), 2nd part. VII. Information systems and access to knowledge.* Paris, UNESCO, 1982.

Annex 3

European Community

The member countries of the European Community are Belgium, Denmark, France, the Federal Republic of Germany, Greece, Ireland, Italy, Luxembourg, the Netherlands, Portugal, Spain and the United Kingdom.

The Commission of the European Communities, advised by the Committee for Information and Documentation on Science and Technology (CIDST), promotes and supports the development of information through programmes and action plans.

The three action plans, run between 1975 and 1983, had several results.

1.   The telecommunication network called EURONET was created for the European Community. EURONET was used by some 2500 organizations for over 100 000 hours during 1985. It uses the packet-switching technology that allows the efficient use of available lines, high quality services and low costs. (For asynchronous terminals the speeds for transmission are 110–1200 bit/s, for synchronous terminals 2400–9600 bit/s.) Since 1985 EURONET has been replaced by an interlinked national public network.

2.   A network of information services called DIANE (Direct Information Access Network for Europe) was launched. DIANE began with 70 data bases on 12 host computers in 1980, and had over 600 data bases on some 60 host computers by 1985. Most important for medicine are the host systems BLAISE, DATA-STAR, DIMDI, ESA-IRS and Télésystèmes Questel. About 85% of the bibliographical data bases can be searched with the DIANE Common Command Language.

3.   A series of sectoral information systems, to cover agricultural, environmental, biomedical and health subjects, was developed and used; in the field of biomedicine the following projects were developed:

— a minimum basic data set within the European Community, starting with essential medical data from hospitals;

— the Pilot Inventory of Biomedical Research Projects (MEDREP);

— an inventory of existing information systems in biomedicine and health care;

— Information Systems on Technical Aids for the Disabled (HANDY-NET) consisting of a set of modules such as HANDYAIDS, an inventory of technical aids; HANDYWHO, an inventory of professional and other groups involved in various ways in technical aids and HANDYSEARCH, an inventory of current research.

The group also has biotechnology projects, such as:

— setting-up of a European data bank on nucleic acid sequences at the European Molecular Biology Laboratory in Heidelberg;

— setting-up of a European Biotechnology Information and Referral Centre at the Science Reference Library in the United Kingdom;

— a study on a preliminary assessment of the feasibility and resource requirements of a computerized European Community information system for microorganism culture collections;

— a study of user needs for information on enzymes and related systems; and

— setting up of a European node at Nice for the hybridoma data bank.

On 27 November 1984, the Council approved a five-year programme (1984–1988) for the development of a specialized information market with two goals. One objective was the improvement of the information environment and market conditions.

The main objective is to improve the use of information products and services of European origin in order to ensure, as far as possible, their economic viability. This is to be achieved by taking appropriate action on existing obstacles, thus resulting in increased user-friendliness and more transparence for information supply and demand.[a]

The other was the reinforcement of the supply and quality of European products and services.

The objective is to create specialized information products and services of European origin which are innovative and unique, and which offer added value with a view to improving the competitiveness of European suppliers on the European and the world markets, as well as their responsiveness to the needs of a wide range of users, thus creating a relative European independence.[a]

Within this programme efforts are actually concentrated on seven *priority areas*: patent information, biotechnology information, materials data banks, information for industry, electronic publishing and image data banks, reducing regional discrepancies and aid to modernizing and linking up of library systems.

---

[a] *Official journal of the European Communities,* No. L 314, 1984.

The European Community will support and encourage efforts leading to advanced information services, such as electronic document delivery and publishing.[a] Based on the results of a call for proposals launched in 1982, the Commission co-financed ten projects, starting in 1984:

— three large-scale experiments in electronic document delivery using different methods of storage such as magnetic disc, microfiche and optical digital disc, transmission such as post, facsimile, wide-band cable, packet-switched network and satellite communication, and ordering such as on-line ordering and video technology;

— seven small- and medium-scale experiments in electronic publishing, among them four electronic journals, one project for on-demand publishing and one project for an electronic invisible college that links a group of experts by microcomputer link over the telephone.

Linguistic problems will remain one of the crucial subjects of the programme and include the development and perfection of multilingual tools such as thesauri, orientation and access services to multilingual information, and automatic translation services.

Through another call for proposals, launched in 1985, the Commission will co-finance some 25 projects referring to the application of new information technologies in the fields of electronic publishing, information for industry and biotechnology.

[a] *Vernimb, C. & Mastroddi, F.* The CEC experiments on electronic document delivery and electronic publishing. *In: International On-line Information Meeting, London, 6–8 December 1983.* Oxford, Learned Information, 1983, pp. 119–130.

Annex 4

Council for Mutual Economic Assistance (CMEA)

The member countries of CMEA are Bulgaria, Cuba, Czechoslovakia, the German Democratic Republic, Hungary, Mongolia, Poland, Romania, the USSR and Viet Nam.

The establishment of the International System of Scientific-Technical Information (ISSTI) is an element of the CMEA complex programme. Its aim is to provide people in the participating countries with complete access to the scientific and technical information of the world. To achieve this goal, ISSTI promotes cooperation between national information systems, the development of international branch-oriented information systems (MOSNTI) and international specialized information systems for the different types of document (MSIS), and the activities of the International Centre for Scientific-Technical Information in Moscow.

ISSTI works through the international division of labour. Standards and norms ensure that uniform methods, technology and techniques are used by the participating countries. The transition to automated information processes is taking place step by step. Some subsystems have been automated already. In the next few years a communications network will be established, which will allow for on-line access to all data bases in the CMEA countries.

The International Centre for Scientific-Technical Information in Moscow is subordinate to the Committee of Authorized Representatives of the ten member countries and does scientific work along with developing ISSTI. It also provides scientific information. For example, it is responsible for the data base on technical reports (MSIS NIR) that documents the technical reports and dissertations produced in the member countries. The information in this data base is recorded on tapes as well as in an abstract journal. Tapes of international data bases such as Science Citation Index, Conference Paper Index and INIS are also available on the computer of the International Centre for Scientific-Technical Information. The international specialized information systems collect, index and disseminate information from one type of document. The information service consists of a tape service, the selective dissemination of information, retrospective searches, bibliographies, abstracts and the provision of copies.

The following MSIS systems function at present:

— MSIS technical reports;

— International Information System for Published Documents (MISOD), identical with the ASSISTENT system;

— MSIS for company catalogues;

— International Patent Information System of the CMEA Member Countries;

— International Information Service for Scientific and Technical Translations;

— International Information System for Scientific-Technical Cinema Films; and

— International Automated System for Registering Serials.

The international branch information systems collect, index and disseminate information on all types of document according to the principle of disciplines or branches. They disseminate complex information to the people who use them. In addition to tape services, selective dissemination of information, retrospective searches and the provision of copies, the supply of synthesized and factual information will become more important. At present, 23 systems (MOSNTI) are being developed, among them the International System for Medical Scientific Information (MEDINFORM).

MEDINFORM is intended to supply complex and complete information to the people who use it. This will be done not only by retrieving scientific documents through the selective dissemination of information, retrospective searches and bibliographies and supplying documents, but also, and increasingly, by providing synthesized and factual information.

Part of this information is collected, indexed and stored by MEDINFORM itself. MEDINFORM has its own classification scheme and a thesaurus of about 11 000 hierarchically ordered descriptors for this purpose. The classification terms and the thesaurus are written and can be used in Russian since Russian is the working language of the ISSTI, and in the national languages of the member countries. Biomedical literature is indexed and abstracted in the different member countries. The resulting tapes are accumulated in a computer centre in Sofia and sent back to the national information centres to be used to provide information services on a national scale.

The present services offered by MEDINFORM are:

— the data base MEDIK with about 40 000 articles annually from periodicals of the member countries, whose tapes are used mainly for the selective dissemination of information, although on-line access is planned;

— the Index Medico Juridicus covering the national literature of CMEA countries on medical law, legal instructions and norms of the public health systems;

— the data base MEDPERIODIK registering national and international biomedical journals and their location in the member countries; and

— the use of such international automated information systems as MEDLINE in Czechoslovakia, German Democratic Republic, Hungary and Poland, Excerpta Medica in Czechoslovakia and the USSR, BIOSIS in Bulgaria and the USSR, as well as Science Citation Index, Conference Paper Index, INIS and others.

Annex 5

Acronyms, abbreviations and titles

This list is limited to items appearing more than once in the text. Names of United Nations organizations such as WHO, ILO and UNESCO are not included. For details on data bases, see Annex 6.

ABDA	Data base on drugs, Bundesvereinigung Deutscher Apothekerverbände
ADONIS	Article Delivery over Network Information Systems
ADRS	Automatic Document Request Service
AGRIS	International information system for the agricultural sciences and technology
AIS	Automated information systems
AIS SIRENA	AIS in CNIMZ
APOLLO	Article Procurement with On-line Ordering (EEC)
ARTEMIS	Automated Retrieval of Text from Europe's Multinational Information Services (EEC)
ASSISTENT	Avtomatizirovannaja spravočno-informacionnaja sistema po nauke i tehnike [Automatized reference-information system for science and technology], VINITI data base
AVLINE	Audovisuals on-line data base
BIOETHICSLINE	Data base on ethics, NLM
BIOMED	*see* LIST-BIOMED — Union list of periodicals in Scandinavia
BIOSIS	Biology and biosciences data base
BIRD	Base d'Information Robert Debré (Centre international pour l'Enfance, France)
BITS	BIOSIS Information Transfer
BLAISE	British Library Automated Information Service
BLLD	British Library Lending Division

BMA	British Medical Association
BRS	Bibliographic Retrieval Services, Inc. (computer host)
CADIST	Centre automatisé de Documentation et d'Information scientifique et technique, France
CAN/SDI	Canadian Selective Dissemination of Information
CANCEREXPRESS	Data base on cancer research, National Cancer Institute, USA
CANCERLIT	Data base on cancer literature, National Cancer Institute, USA
CANCERNET	Data base on cancer research, Institut Gustave Roussy, France and DKFZ
CANCERPROJ	Data base on cancer research, National Cancer Institute, USA
CANDO	Classification alphanumérique pour la Documentation médicale
CAS	Chemical Abstract Service and data base
CIS	Congressional Information Service
CLINPROT	Data base on clinical cancer protocols, National Cancer Institute, USA
CMEA	Council for Mutual Economic Assistance
CMW	Centrum Medyczne Ksztalcenia [Medical Centre for Training], Warsaw (in HECLINET)
CNIMZ	Centr za naučna Informacii pa Medicina i Zdrazeopazvane [Centre for Scientific Information in Medicine and Public Health], Sofia, Bulgaria
CNRS	Centre national de la Recherche scientifique, France
COMPENDEX	Data base on engineering, USA
CONFINDEX/CPI	Data Base on Conference Papers Index, USA
DARE	Data retrieval system for the social sciences and humanities (UNESCO)
DATA-STAR	Host, based in Switzerland
DBMIST	Division des Bibliothèques et Musées et de l'Information scientifique et technique
DEVSIS	Development of Science Information Systems (UNESCO)
DHSS	Department of Health and Social Security
DIALOG	Dialog Information Services, Inc.
DIANE	Direct Information Access Network for Europe, *see* EURONET

DIMDI	Deutsches Institut für medizinische Dokumentation und Information, Cologne, Federal Republic of Germany
DKFZ	Deutsches Krebsforschungszentrum, Heidelberg, Federal Republic of Germany
DKI	Deutsches Krankenhausinstitut, Düsseldorf, Federal Republic of Germany
DOBIS/LIBIS	Data base of ISS, Italy
DOR	Differencirovannoje Obespečenije Rukovad'vo [Selected Management Information Service], VINITI
DSI	Dansk Sygehus Institut [Danish Hospital Institute], Copenhagen, Denmark
EDP	Electronic data processing
EEC	European Economic Community
EMBASE	Excerpta Medica data base
EPOS/VIRA	Swedish data host
ERIC	Educational Resources Information Center data base
ESA/IRS	European Space Agency information retrieval system
ESKOM	Edina Sistema za Kommandiroviskite [Unified Information Command System], VINITI
EURONET	Communication network of the EEC — ceased bearing that name in 1985
FRANCIS	Fichier de Recherches automatisées sur les Nouveautés, la Communication et l'Information en Sciences sociales et humaines (data base of Télésystèmes QUESTEL)
FSTA	Foods Science and Technology Abstracts and data base
G-CAM	French host and server
GCNMB	Gosudarstvennaja Central'naja Naučnaja Medicinskaja Biblioteka [State Central Scientific and Medical Library], Moscow, USSR
GRIPS	General Relation-based Information Processing System, see DIMDI
GSNTI	Gosudarstvennaja Sistema Naučno-Tehničeskoj Informacii [State System for Scientific and Technical Information], Moscow, USSR
HEALTH	Data base on health planning and administration, NLM, USA

93

HECLINET	Health Care Literature Information Network (and data base)
HELLIS	Health Literature and Library Information Services (WHO)
HISTLINE	Data base on history of medicine, NLM, USA
HORIZONT	Data base in CNIMZ
HSELINE	Data base on Health and Safety Executive on-line, United Kingdom
IARC	International Agency for Research on Cancer, Lyon, France
ICRD-BP	International Cancer Research Data Bank Program, IARC
IDIS	Institut für Dokumentation und Information über Sozialmedizin und öffentliches Gesundheitswesen, Bielefeld, Federal Republic of Germany
IDIS-SOMED	IDIS-Sozial Medizin, data base of IDIS on social medicine
IFK	Institut für Krankenhausbau, Berlin (West)
IMA	Information médicale automatisée
IMD	Institut für maschinelle Dokumentation, Graz, Austria
INION	Institut Naučnoj Informacii po Obščestvennym Naukam [Institute for Scientific Information for the Social Sciences], Moscow, USSR
INIS	International Nuclear Information System data base, International Atomic Energy Agency
INSERM	Institut national de la Santé et de la Recherche médicale, Paris, France
INSPEC	Information Services for the Physics and Engineering Communities — data base, United Kingdom
INTERNIST	Data base of VINITI
IPA	International Pharmaceutical Abstracts, United Kingdom
IRCS	International Research Communications System
ISI	Institute for Scientific Information, Philadelphia, USA
ISI/BIOMED	Data base of ISI
ISORID	International Information System of Research in Documentation
ISS	Istituto Superiore di Sanità, Rome, Italy

ISSTI	International System of Scientific and Technical Information (CMEA)
ITOGI	Automated information system of VINITI on research
IWIM	Institut für Wissenschaftsinformation in der Medizin, Berlin, German Democratic Republic
KIBIC	Karolinska Institutets Bibliotek og Informationscentralen [Library and Information Centre of the Karolinska Institute], Stockholm, Sweden
LIBRIS	Library information system (Italy)
MARC	Machine readable cataloguing
MEDIK	Medicinskaja informacija [Medical information], MEDINFORM data base
MEDINFORM	Medical information system (CMEA)
MEDLARS	Medical Literature Analysis and Retrieval System and data base
MEDLINE	MEDLARS on-line
MEDPERIODIK	Medicinskaja periodika [Medical periodicals], data base in VINITI
MeSH	Medical subject headings (MEDLINE thesaurus)
MIC	Medicinska Information Centralen [Medical Information Centre], Stockholm, Sweden
MIDIST	Mission interministérielle de l'Information scientifique et technique, France
MISOD	Meždunarodnaja Informacionnaja Sistema po Opublikovannym Dokumentam [International Information System for Published Documents — ASSISTENT q.v.]
MOSNTI	Meždunarodnaja Otraslevaja Sistema Naučno-Tehničeskoj Informacii [International Branch System for Medico-Technical Information], VINITI
MSIS	Meždunarodnaja Specializirovannaja Informacionnaja Sistema [International Specialized Information System], primary information data base of CMEA
MSIS NIR	Meždunarodnaja Specializirovannaja Informacionnaja Sistema po Naučno-Issledovatelskim Rabotam [International Specialized Information System on Scientific Research Work]
NATIS	National infrastructures of information (UNESCO)
NHS	National Health Service (United Kingdom)

NIMR	National Institute for Medical Research (United Kingdom)
NLM	National Library of Medicine, USA
OASNMI	Otraslevaja Avtomatizirovannaja Sistema Naučnoj Medicinskoj Informacii [Branch Automated System for Scientific Medical Information], Moscow, USSR
ÖBIG	Österreichisches Bundesinstitut für Gesundheitswesen, Vienna, Austria
OCLC	On-line Computer Library Center
PASCAL	Programme appliqué à la Sélection et à la Compilation automatique de la Littérature, data base, France
PESTDOC	Pesticidal literature documentation data base
POPLINE	Population problems data base, NLM
PRE-MED	Data base of BRS
PRIME	Minicomputer used in DHSS
PSYCINFO	Psychological Abstracts information service and data base
PSYNDEX	Psychologischer Index
QUESTEL	French support telesystem
RESHUS	Réseau d'Information en Sciences humaines de la Santé, France
RINGDOC	Pharmaceutical literature documentation data base
RTECS	Registry of Toxic Effects of Chemical Substances, data base, USA
SCANNET	Scandinavian network
SCI	Science Citation Index
SCICON	United Kingdom host
SDI	Selective dissemination of information
SIGLE	System for Information on Grey Literature (EEC)
SIRENA	AIS developed by CNIMZ
SKI	Schweizerisches Krankenhausinstitut, Aarau, Switzerland
SPINES	Science and Technology Policies Information Exchange System (UNESCO)
SPRI	Sjukvardens och Socialvardens Planerings- och Rationaliseringsinstitut [Institute for Planning and Rationalization of Health and Social Care], Stockholm, Sweden

STATUS	Software used on PRIME
TDB	Toxicology Data Bank
TELEGENLINE	Genetic technology data base
TELENET	Telephone communication network
TOXLINE	Toxicology information on-line data base
TRANSINDEX	Scientific and technical translation data base
TYMNET	International telephone communication network
UNAFORMEC	Union nationale des Associations de Formation médicale continue
UNISIST	Universal system for information in science and technology
VCP	Vsesojuzny Centr Perevodov [All-Union Centre for Translations], Moscow, USSR
VESKA	Verband Schweizerischer Krankenhausanstalten, Switzerland
VINITI	Vsesojuzny Institut Naučnoj i Tehničeskoj Informacii [All-Union Institute for Scientific and Technical Information], Moscow, USSR
VNIIMI	Vsesojuzny Naučno-Issledovatel'skij Institut Medicinskoj i Mediko-Tehničeskoj Informacii [All-Union Scientific-Technical Institute in Medical and Technical Information], Moscow, USSR
VNIIPI	Vsejojuznij Naučno-Issledovatel'skij Institut Patentnoj Informacij [All-Union Scientific-Technical Institute on Patents Information], Moscow, USSR
VNTICENTR	Vsesojuznij Naučnoj-Tehničeskij Informacionnij Centr [All-Union Centre for Scientific-Technical Information], Moscow, USSR
WHODOC	WHO documents (selection)
WPI	World Patents Index data base
ZBM	Zentralbibliothek der Medizin, Cologne, Federal Republic of Germany
ZDB	Zeitschrift Databank, Berlin (West)

Annex 6

Main health-related data bases

ABDA Factual data on active ingredients of drugs; 10 000 drugs registered in the Federal Republic of Germany, and interactions between drugs
Originator: ABDA/DIMDI
On-line printed version access (part or whole): 1966–

ASSISTENT Multidisciplinary; 16 000 journals (biosciences 5000); 1.5 million citations per year (biosciences 300 000)
Originator: VINITI
On-line printed version access (part or whole): *Referativnij žurnal*

AVLINE Audiovisual materials; about 11 000 citations
Originator: NLM
On-line printed version access (part or whole): 1975–

BIOETHICSLINE Ethics and public policy in health care and research; about 62 000 citations plus 4500 per year
Originator: NLM
On-line printed version access (part or whole): 1973–

BIOSIS Biology and biosciences; 8500 journals; about 3.5 million citations plus 300 000 per year
Originator: Biosciences Information Service, USA
On-line printed version access (part or whole): 1970–, *Biological abstracts*

BIRD Base d'Informations Robert Debré — family and childhood (0–20 years); about 60 000 citations plus 15 000 per year
Originator: Centre international de l'Enfance, France
On-line printed version access (part or whole): 1981–, *Courrier de l'enfance*

CANCEREXPRESS	Recent key articles on cancer research; 10 000 citations **Originator**: National Cancer Institute, USA **On-line printed version access (part or whole)**: latest 4 months
CANCERLIT	Cancer literature; 450 000 citations plus 50 000 per year **Originator**: National Cancer Institute, USA **On-line printed version access (part or whole)**: 1963–
CANCERNET	Cancer research; 1100 journals; 30 000 citations plus 12 000 per year **Originator**: Institut Gustave Roussy, France and DKFZ **On-line printed version access (part or whole)**: 1968–
CANCERPROJ	Cancer research projects (unpublished); predominantly USA plus 50 other countries; 21 000 descriptions **Originator**: National Cancer Institute, USA **On-line printed version access (part or whole)**: 1978–1981
CAS	Chemistry and biochemistry; 14 000 journals; about 5.5 million citations plus 500 000 per year **Originator**: Chemical Abstracts Services, USA **On-line printed version access (part or whole)**: 1969–, *Chemical abstracts*
CLINPROT	Clinical cancer protocols; about 4300 protocols **Originator**: National Cancer Institute, USA **On-line printed version access (part or whole)**: 1977–
COMPENDEX	Engineering and related areas; 1 million citations plus 10 000 per year **Originator**: Engineering Index, Inc., USA **On-line printed version access (part or whole)**: 1969–, *Engineering index*
CONFINDEX/CPI	Conference Papers Index: items presented at scientific/technical meetings; 1 million citations plus 100 000 per year **Originator**: Data Courier, USA **On-line printed version access (part or whole)**: 1973–, *Conference papers index*
EMBASE	Excerpta Medica data base, covering general field of biomedicine; more emphasis on Europe than MEDLARS; 4000 journals; about 2.2 million citations plus 250 000 per year **Originator**: Excerpta Medica, Netherlands **On-line printed version access (part or whole)**: 1974–, *Excerpta medica*

ERIC	Educational Resources Information Center; 470 000 citations plus 38 000 per year **Originator**: National Institute of Education, USA **On-line printed version access (part or whole)**: 1966–, *Resources in education*
FSTA	Food science and technology; 250 000 citations plus 20 000 per year **Originator**: International Food Information Services, Reading University, United Kingdom **On-line printed version access (part or whole)**: 1969–, *Food science and technology abstracts*
HEALTH	Health planning and administration, and non-clinical aspects of health care delivery; including Hospital Literature Index, Nursing Index; about 300 000 citations plus 25 000 per year **Originator**: NLM **On-line printed version access (part or whole)**: 1975–
HECLINET	Hospital administration, non-clinical aspects of health care delivery and hospital management; Denmark, Federal Republic of Germany, Sweden, Switzerland; about 60 000 citations plus 4500 per year **Originator**: IFK and DKI **On-line printed version access (part or whole)**: 1969–, *Hospital literature index*
HISTLINE	History of medicine; about 75 000 citations plus 10 000 per year **Originator**: NLM **On-line printed version access (part or whole)**: 1970–
HSELINE	Health and safety (environment and occupation); about 40 000 citations plus 7000 per year **Originator**: Health and Safety Executive, United Kingdom **On-line printed version access (part or whole)**: 1977–
INIS	Nuclear science; about 300 000 citations plus 75 000 per year **Originator**: International Atomic Energy Agency **On-line printed version access (part or whole)**: 1970–, *INIS atomindex*
INSPEC	Physics, electrical and electronic developments, and computers; about 2 million citations plus 160 000 per year **Originator**: Institution of Electrical Engineers **On-line printed version access (part or whole)**: 1971–, *Physics abstracts; electrical abstracts; Computer and control abstracts*

IPA	International Pharmaceutical Abstracts; 700 journals; about 70 000 citations plus 7000 per year **Originator**: American Society of Hospital Pharmacists **On-line printed version access (part or whole)**: 1970–, *International pharmaceutical abstracts*
MEDIK	Medicinskaja Informacija, covering general field of biomedicine; literature of CMEA countries; 320 journals; about 100 000 citations plus 35 000 per year **Originator**: MEDINFORM
MEDLARS	Medical Literature Analysis and Retrieval System; biomedicine; 3200 journals; about 4.5 million citations **Originator**: NLM **On-line printed version access (part or whole)**: 1964–, *Index medicus*
PASCAL	Programme appliqué à la Sélection et à la Compilation automatique de la Littérature; 13 000 journals; about 5 million citations plus 500 000 per year **Originator**: CNRS **On-line printed version access (part or whole)**: 1979–, *Bulletin signalétique*
PESTDOC	Pesticides literature; about 130 000 citations plus 10 000 per year **Originator**: Derwent, United Kingdom **On-line printed version access (part or whole)**: 1968–, *PestDoc abstracts journal*
POPLINE	Population and family planning problems, including law and policy issues; about 130 000 citations plus 12 000 per year **Originator**: NLM **On-line printed version access (part or whole)**: 1970–
PSYCINFO	Psychology; about 2.2 million citations plus 250 000 per year **Originator**: American Psychological Association **On-line printed version access (part or whole)**: 1967–, *Psychological abstracts*
RINGDOC	Pharmaceutical literature documentation **Originator**: Derwent, United Kingdom **On-line printed version access (part or whole)**: 1976–, *Ringdoc abstracts journal*
RTECS	Registry of Toxic Effects of Chemical Substances; 67 000 substances **Originator**: National Institute of Occupational Safety and Health, USA **On-line printed version access (part or whole)**: 1979–

TELEGENLINE	Genetic technology; about 15 000 citations plus 3500 per year **Originator**: Environmental Information Center, USA **On-line printed version access (part or whole)**: 1973–, *Telegen reporter*
TOXLINE	Toxicology information on-line, toxicology studies, analysis of chemical substances **Originator**: NLM **On-line printed version access (part or whole)**: 1965–, *Chemical biological activities abstracts on health effects of environmental pollutants; International pharmaceutical abstracts; Toxicity bibliography; Pesticides abstracts*
TRANSINDEX/WTI	Scientific and technical translation index; about 150 000 plus 30 000 per year **Originator**: CNRS, France and International Translations Centre, Delft, Netherlands **On-line printed version access (part or whole)**: 1978–, *World transindex*
WPI	Patents index for 24 countries and for Europe as a whole; over 1 million patents plus 245 000 per year **Originator**: Derwent, United Kingdom **On-line printed version access (part or whole)**: 1963–, *World patent index; Central patent index*